I0063579

Nutrition and the Function of the Central Nervous System

Nutrition and the Function of the Central Nervous System

Special Issue Editor

Billy R. Hammond

MDPI • Basel • Beijing • Wuhan • Barcelona • Belgrade

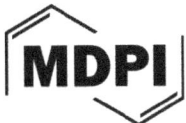

MDPI

Special Issue Editor
Billy R. Hammond
University of Georgia
USA

Editorial Office
MDPI
St. Alban-Anlage 66
Basel, Switzerland

This is a reprint of articles from the Special Issue published online in the open access journal *Nutrients* (ISSN 2072-6643) from 2017 to 2018 (available at: http://www.mdpi.com/journal/nutrients/special_issues/nutri_cns)

For citation purposes, cite each article independently as indicated on the article page online and as indicated below:

LastName, A.A.; LastName, B.B.; LastName, C.C. Article Title. *Journal Name* **Year**, *Article Number*, Page Range.

ISBN 978-3-03897-051-4 (Pbk)
ISBN 978-3-03897-052-1 (PDF)

Articles in this volume are Open Access and distributed under the Creative Commons Attribution (CC BY) license, which allows users to download, copy and build upon published articles even for commercial purposes, as long as the author and publisher are properly credited, which ensures maximum dissemination and a wider impact of our publications. The book taken as a whole is © 2018 MDPI, Basel, Switzerland, distributed under the terms and conditions of the Creative Commons license CC BY-NC-ND (http://creativecommons.org/licenses/by-nc-nd/4.0/).

Contents

About the Special Issue Editor

Billy R. Hammond is a full Professor in the Brain and Behavioral Sciences program at the University of Georgia (UGA). He is also faculty in the Foods and Nutrition and Gerontology program at UGA and the Principal Investigator of the Vision Sciences Laboratory. The Vision Sciences laboratory at the University of Georgia studies all aspects of the human visual system. This extends from basic studies of the cornea, lens and retina to applied studies of visual processing within the brain. A primary focus of the laboratory has been the investigation of how lifestyle, primarily dietary, influences both the development of degenerative disease and the normal function of the central nervous system. For example, we have published numerous studies, including some examples contained in the current volume, on how the dietary carotenoids lutein and zeaxanthin within the fovea (termed macular pigment or the macula lutea) relate to various aspects of retinal and brain function

Preface to "Nutrition and the Function of the Central Nervous System"

This volume is focused on the role of nutrition in the development and maintenance of the central nervous system (CNS, primarily retina and brain). This focus encompasses both nutritional effects on normal function and the prevention and treatment of CNS disease. The critical role of diet in most bodily systems (such as the cardiovascular or skeletal system) and in the prevention of disease (e.g., metabolic conditions, such as acquired diabetes) is largely accepted as an axiom. It is only relatively recently, however, that researchers, particularly neuroscientists, began to focus on how diet influences the very organ system that is at the center of our self, the brain. The retina is the most metabolically active tissue in the body and is impacted early by metabolic diseases such as diabetes. The brain is some 2% of our mass, but about 20–25% of inspired oxygen is delivered to this highly vascularized fatty (some 60% by volume) tissue. The CNS is not simply influenced by diet, it is built from, maintained, and preserved by diet. This premise is explored in this Special Issue.

For example, in one group of papers from the University of Georgia and the University of Illinois, Urbana Champagn, researchers explore the role of lutein on brain function. Lutein is a phytopigment that is obtained from green leafy vegetables and is concentrated in key areas of the brain involved in higher cognitive function, such as prefrontal cortex and hippocampus. Using classic cognitive and neuroimaging methods, and central nervous system biomarkers of lutein (MPOD), the researchers examine how lutein influences brain function in both adults and children. This volume also includes work based on animal models that explore how diet affects other aspects of nervous system function, such as hyperalgesia, and basic work on the gut microbiome and inflammation.

Billy R. Hammond
Special Issue Editor

nutrients

MDPI

Communication

The Gut Microbial Metabolite Trimethylamine-*N*-Oxide Is Present in Human Cerebrospinal Fluid

Daniele Del Rio [1], Francesca Zimetti [1], Paolo Caffarra [2], Michele Tassotti [1], Franco Bernini [1], Furio Brighenti [1], Andrea Zini [3] and Ilaria Zanotti [1,*]

[1] Dipartimento di Scienze degli Alimenti e del Farmaco, Università degli Studi di Parma,
Parco Area delle Scienze 27/A, 43124 Parma, Italy; daniele.delrio@unipr.it (D.D.R.);
francesca.zimetti@unipr.it (F.Z.); michele.tassotti@studenti.unipr.it (M.T.); f.bernini@unipr.it (Fr.B.);
furio.brighenti@unipr.it (Fu.B.)

[2] Dipartimento di Medicina e Chirurgia, Unità di Neuroscienze, Università degli Studi di Parma,
via Gramsci 14, 43126 Parma, Italy; paolo.caffarra@unipr.it

[3] Dipartimento di Neuroscienze, Nuovo Ospedale Civile "S.Agostino-Estense",
Azienda Ospedaliera Universitaria, via Giardini 1355, 41100 Modena, Italy; andrea.zini@me.com

* Correspondence: ilaria.zanotti@unipr.it; Tel.: +39-0521-905-040

Received: 18 August 2017; Accepted: 20 September 2017; Published: 22 September 2017

Abstract: Trimethylamine-*N*-oxide (TMAO) is a small organic molecule, derived from the intestinal and hepatic metabolism of dietary choline and carnitine. Although the involvement of TMAO in the framework of many chronic diseases has been recently described, no evidence on its putative role in the central nervous system has been provided. The aim of this study was to evaluate whether TMAO is present at detectable levels in human cerebrospinal fluid (CSF). CSF was collected for diagnostic purposes from 58 subjects by lumbar puncture and TMAO was quantified by using liquid chromatography coupled with multiple-reaction monitoring mass spectrometry. The molecule was detected in all samples, at concentrations ranging between 0.11 and 6.43 μmol/L. Further analysis on CSF revealed that a total of 22 subjects were affected by Alzheimer's disease (AD), 16 were affected by non-AD related dementia, and 20 were affected by other neurological disorders. However, the stratification of TMAO levels according to the neurological diagnoses revealed no differences among the three groups. In conclusion, we provide the first evidence that TMAO can be assessed in human CSF, but the actual impact of this dietary metabolite in the patho-physiolgy of the central nervous system requires further study.

Keywords: trimethylamine-*N*-oxide; gut microbiota; central nervous system

1. Introduction

It is now generally accepted that gut microbiota represents a major regulator of health and disease in humans, both contributing to the host metabolic and immune functions and potentially driving the onset of chronic diseases [1]. Among the mechanisms accounting for the pathological implications of the microbiota, the metabolism of dietary-derived products is currently a matter of wide interest. As an example, the ingestion of food rich in choline (dairy products, eggs, fish) or carnitine (red meat) is associated with increased plasma levels of trimethylamine-*N*-oxide (TMAO) through the sequential action of intestinal microbes and the hepatic flavin monooxigenase 3 (FMO3) [2]. This small organic molecule has drawn the attention of the scientific world following the demonstration that high plasma levels are associated with an increased risk of cardiovascular events [3–5]. Whereas the existence of a reciprocal influence between gut and brain is not a matter of debate, no evidence of clinical implications of TMAO in the central nervous system has yet been documented. In order to address this issue, we assessed TMAO in cerebrospinal fluid (CSF) collected from 58 subjects that underwent a lumbar puncture for diagnostic purposes and demonstrate for the first time that TMAO is present at detectable levels in the central nervous system.

2. Materials and Methods

CSF were obtained at the Neurology Unit of the University of Parma for diagnostic purposes after informed consent. The study was approved by The Institutional Review Board of the University of Parma (authorization number 0058/2017). Samples were collected in the morning, after one night of fasting, and immediately stored at −80 °C.

For TMAO quantification, before the analysis, each sample was added with TMAO-d9 as internal standard and then extracted with acidified acetonitrile, as previously described [6]. Samples were centrifuged and the supernatants collected and analyzed by a UHPLC DIONEX Ultimate 3000 equipped with a triple quadrupole TSQ Vantage (Thermo Fisher Scientific Inc., San Josè, CA, USA) fitted with a heated-ESI (H-ESI) (Thermo Fisher Scientific Inc., San Jose, CA, USA) probe. Separations were carried out by means of an XBridge BEH HILIC XP (100 mm × 2.1 mm) column, with a 2.5 μm particle size (Waters, Milford, MA, USA). Statistical analyses were performed using Prism 6.0 (GraphPad Inc., San Diego, CA, USA).

Alzheimer's Disease (AD) (n = 22) and non-AD related dementia (non-AD) (n = 16) was diagnosed according to International Working Group (IWG)-2 criteria [7]. Non-AD includes frontotemporal dementia, corticobasal degeneration, and degenerative Parkinsonism. Aβ 1-42, tau, and phospho-tau levels were evaluated via enzyme-linked immunosorbent assay (ELISA) (Fujirebio, Ghent, Belgium). The third group included age- and sex-matched subjects that experienced neurological disorders unrelated to demyelinating inflammatory disorders, stroke, and neurodegenerative and infective diseases.

3. Results

All tested samples showed detectable amounts of TMAO, in a range between 0.11 and 6.43 μmol/L (median: 0.665 μmol/L, 95% CI-0.490 to 0.870 μmol/L) (Figure 1).

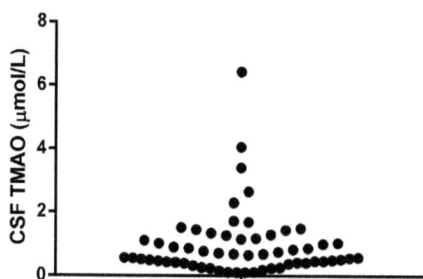

Figure 1. Trimethylamine-*N*-oxide (TMAO) concentrations in human cerebrospinal fluid (CSF). TMAO was quantified as described in the method section.

Successively, the data were stratified according to the neurological diagnoses following the analysis of CSF. Demographic data and dementia diagnostic parameters of subjects are shown in Table 1.

Table 1. Demographic data and dementia diagnostic parameters.

	AD (*n* = 22)	Non-AD (*n* = 16)	Other Neurological Disorders (*n* = 20)
Age (years)	69 ± 9	63 ± 8	65 ± 17
Male sex, *n* (%)	12 (54)	9 (56)	10 (50)
Aβ 1–42 (ng/L)	416 (177–674)	675 *** (288–1540)	N.E.
Tau (ng/L)	449 (109–1644)	204 *** (22–564)	N.E.
Phospo-Tau (ng/L)	80 (25–742)	33 *** (3–64)	N.E.
TMAO (µmol/L)	0.520 (0.32–1.15)	0.710, (0.56–1.50)	0.570, (0.42–1.00)

Data are expressed as mean ± S.D. for normally distributed values or as median (interquartile range) for data that are not normally distributed. The one way ANOVA test was applied to compare the three groups for age; the non-parametric two-tailed Mann Whitney test was applied to compare AD and non-AD subjects for CSF neurobiomarkers. *** $p < 0.01$ vs. AD. AD: Alzheimer's disease; non-AD: non-AD related dementia. N.E.: not evaluated.

As expected, patients with prodromal AD had significantly decreased Aβ 1-42 and increased tau and phospho-tau in CSF compared to non-AD subjects.

No differences in the actual concentrations of TMAO were observed among the three groups (one-way ANOVA $p = 0.326$).

4. Discussion

TMAO has been recently proposed as a novel prognostic marker of cardiovascular events, given the association of its plasma levels with indexes of atherosclerotic plaque vulnerability [8], major cardiac events [5], and death [9]. Similarly, it has been associated with other chronic diseases, such as diabetes [10] and cancer [11], further strengthening the pathological implications of this microbiota metabolite.

The recognized connections between gut and brain has recently piqued interest in the impact of diet and microbiota on the functionality of the central nervous system. Up to now, only one work on lactic acid and short chain fatty acids have revealed how dietary-derived products may exert (potentially adverse) neurological effects [12].

The present study originates from the hypothesis that TMAO may play a direct role in the central nervous system. As a preliminary, fundamental aspect, its presence in the CSF needed to be assessed, and this was the main aim of this short study. A recent work, based on an innovative microphysiology system hypothesized that TMAO could cross the blood–brain barrier [13], but this has never been demonstrated in vivo. For the first time, TMAO has been measured in human CSF, reaching quantifiable levels in all tested samples. Unfortunately, plasma samples from the same subjects were not available, preventing any correlation analysis between biological fluids. Published data from large epidemiological studies revealed that TMAO in plasma may fluctuate in a very wide range of concentrations (0.08–250 µmol/L) and that it is affected by several factors, including dietary intake of choline and carnitine-containing food, the composition of microbiota, and the activity of FMO3 [2]. The levels we detected are consistent with the hypothesis that a small fraction of liver-derived TMAO can cross the blood–brain barrier, but we cannot rule out that a fraction of the TMAO detected in CSF may derive from de novo synthesis, as expression of FMO3 has been detected in the adult brain [14].

In the small tested group of subjects, TMAO levels in CSF are apparently unrelated to the diagnosed neurological disorders. However, establishing the prognostic value of TMAO is beyond the scope of this study, so it is not yet possible to draw conclusions on this aspect.

Albeit preliminary, this study introduces an interesting scenario about the actual role of TMAO in modulating functions of the central nervous system. Future studies in proper in vitro and in vivo models will address this issue, adding novel pieces to the gut–brain axis puzzle.

Acknowledgments: This work was partially funded by University of Parma core funding (FIL 2014-2017).

Author Contributions: I.Z. and A.Z. conceived and designed the experiments; P.C. and M.T. performed the experiments; D.D.R. and F.Z. analyzed the data; I.Z. and D.D.R. wrote the paper; F.Bernini and F.Brighenti critically reviewed the paper.

Conflicts of Interest: The authors declare no conflict of interest.

References

1. Lynch, S.V.; Pedersen, O. The human intestinal microbiome in health and disease. *N. Engl. J. Med.* **2016**, *375*, 2369–2379. [CrossRef] [PubMed]
2. Cho, C.E.; Caudill, M.A. Trimethylamine-*N*-oxide: Friend, foe, or simply caught in the cross-fire? *Trends Endocrinol. Metab.* **2017**, *28*, 121–130. [CrossRef] [PubMed]
3. Senthong, V.; Li, X.S.; Hudec, T.; Coughlin, J.; Wu, Y.; Levison, B.; Wang, Z.; Hazen, S.L.; Tang, W.H.W. Plasma trimethylamine *N*-oxide, a gut microbe-generated phosphatidylcholine metabolite, is associated with atherosclerotic burden. *J. Am. Coll. Cardiol.* **2016**, *67*, 2620–2628. [CrossRef] [PubMed]
4. Suzuki, T.; Heaney, L.M.; Jones, D.J.L.; Ng, L.L. Trimethylamine *N*-oxide and risk stratification after acute myocardial infarction. *Clin. Chem.* **2017**, *63*, 420–428. [CrossRef] [PubMed]
5. Li, X.S.; Obeid, S.; Klingenberg, R.; Gencer, B.; Mach, F.; Raber, L.; Windecker, S.; Rodondi, N.; Nanchen, D.; Muller, O.; et al. Gut microbiota-dependent trimethylamine *N*-oxide in acute coronary syndromes: A prognostic marker for incident cardiovascular events beyond traditional risk factors. *Eur. Heart J.* **2017**, *38*, 1–11. [CrossRef] [PubMed]
6. Miller, C.A.; Corbin, K.D.; Costa, K.; Zhang, S.; Zhao, X.; Galanko, J.A.; Blevins, T.; Bennett, B.J.; Connor, A.O.; Zeisel, S.H. Effect of egg ingestion on trimethylamine-*N*-oxide production in humans: A randomized, controlled, dose-response study. *Am. J. Clin. Nutr.* **2014**, *100*, 778–786. [CrossRef] [PubMed]
7. Dubois, B.; Feldman, H.H.; Jacova, C.; Hampel, H.; Molinuevo, J.L.; Blennow, K.; Dekosky, S.T.; Gauthier, S.; Selkoe, D.; Bateman, R.; et al. Advancing research diagnostic criteria for Alzheimer's disease: The IWG-2 criteria. *Lancet Neurol.* **2014**, *13*, 614–629. [CrossRef]
8. Fu, Q.; Zhao, M.; Wang, D.; Hu, H.; Guo, C.; Chen, W.; Li, Q.; Zheng, L.; Chen, B. Coronary plaque characterization assessed by optical coherence tomography and plasma trimethylamine-*N*-oxide levels in patients with coronary artery disease. *Am. J. Cardiol.* **2016**, *118*, 1311–1315. [CrossRef] [PubMed]
9. Senthong, V.; Wang, Z.; Fan, Y.; Wu, Y.; Hazen, S.L.; Tang, W.H.W. Trimethylamine *N*-oxide and mortality risk in patients with peripheral artery disease. *J. Am. Heart Assoc.* **2016**, *5*, 1–9. [CrossRef] [PubMed]
10. Dambrova, M.; Latkovskis, G.; Kuka, J.; Strele, I.; Konrade, I.; Grinberga, S.; Hartmane, D.; Pugovics, O.; Erglis, A.; Liepinsh, E. Diabetes is associated with higher trimethylamine *N*-oxide plasma levels. *Exp. Clin. Endocrinol. Diabetes* **2016**, *124*, 251–256. [CrossRef] [PubMed]
11. Bae, S.; Ulrich, C.M.; Neuhouser, M.L.; Malysheva, O.; Bailey, L.B.; Xiao, L.; Brown, E.C.; Cushing-Haugen, K.L.; Zheng, Y.; Cheng, T.Y.D.; et al. Plasma choline metabolites and colorectal cancer risk in the women's health initiative observational study. *Cancer Res.* **2014**, *74*, 7442–7452. [CrossRef] [PubMed]
12. Galland, L. The gut microbiome and the brain. *J. Med. Food* **2014**, *17*, 1261–1272. [CrossRef] [PubMed]
13. Vernetti, L.; Gough, A.; Baetz, N.; Blutt, S.; Broughman, J.R.; Brown, J.A.; Foulke-Abel, J.; Hasan, N.; In, J.; Kelly, E.; et al. Functional coupling of human microphysiology systems: Intestine, liver, kidney proximal tubule, blood-brain barrier and skeletal muscle. *Sci. Rep.* **2017**, *7*, 42296. [CrossRef] [PubMed]
14. Cashman, J.R.; Zhang, J. Human flavin-containing monooxygenases. *Annu. Rev. Pharmacol. Toxicol.* **2006**, *46*, 65–100. [CrossRef] [PubMed]

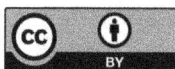

© 2017 by the authors. Licensee MDPI, Basel, Switzerland. This article is an open access article distributed under the terms and conditions of the Creative Commons Attribution (CC BY) license (http://creativecommons.org/licenses/by/4.0/).

nutrients

MDPI

Article

The Food-Specific Serum IgG Reactivity in Major Depressive Disorder Patients, Irritable Bowel Syndrome Patients and Healthy Controls

Hanna Karakula-Juchnowicz [1,2,*], Mirosława Gałęcka [3], Joanna Rog [1,*], Anna Bartnicka [3], Zuzanna Łukaszewicz [3], Pawel Krukow [2], Justyna Morylowska-Topolska [2], Karolina Skonieczna-Zydecka [4], Tomasz Krajka [5], Kamil Jonak [1,6] and Dariusz Juchnowicz [7]

[1]   1st Department of Psychiatry, Psychotherapy and Early Intervention Medical University of Lublin, Gluska Street 1, 20-439 Lublin, Poland; jonak.kamil@gmail.com
[2]   Department of Clinical Neuropsychiatry Medical University of Lublin, Gluska Street 1, 20-439 Lublin, Poland; pawelkrukow@umlub.pl (P.K.); justynamorylowska@op.pl (J.M.-T.)
[3]   Institute of Microecology, Sielska Street 10, 60-129 Poznan, Poland; drgalecka@instytut-mikroekologii.pl (M.G.); anna.bartnicka@instytut-mikroekologii.pl (A.B.); dietetyk@instytut-mikroekologii.pl (Z.L.)
[4]   Department of Biochemistry and Human Nutrition, Pomeranian Medical University in Szczecin, Broniewskiego Street 24, 71-460 Szczecin, Poland, karzyd@pum.edu.pl
[5]   Faculty of Mechanical Engineering, Department of Mathematics, Lublin University of Technology, Nadbystrzycka Street 36, 20-618 Lublin, Poland; t.krajka@pollub.pl
[6]   Department of Biomedical Engineering, Lublin University of Technology, Nadbystrzycka Street 38D, 20-618 Lublin, Poland
[7]   Department of Psychiatric Nursing Medical University of Lublin, Szkolna Street 18, 20-124 Lublin, Poland; juchnowiczdariusz@wp.pl
*   Correspondence: karakula.hanna@gmail.com (H.K.-J.); rog.joann@gmail.com (J.R.)

Received: 2 April 2018; Accepted: 24 April 2018; Published: 28 April 2018

Abstract: There is an increasing amount of evidence which links the pathogenesis of irritable bowel syndrome (IBS) with food IgG hyperreactivity. Some authors have suggested that food IgG hyperreactivity could be also involved in the pathophysiology of major depressive disorder (MDD). The aim of this study was to compare levels of serum IgG against 39 selected food antigens between three groups of participants: patients with MDD (MDD group), patients with IBS (IBS group) and healthy controls (HC group). The study included 65 participants (22 in the MDD group, 22 in the IBS group and 21 in the HC group). Serum IgG levels were examined using enzyme-linked immunosorbent assay (ELISA). Medical records, clinical data and laboratory results were collected for the analysis. IgG food hyperreactivity (interpreted as an average of levels of IgG antibodies above 7.5 µg/mL) was detected in 28 (43%) participants, including 14 (64%) from the MDD group, ten (46%) from the IBS group and four (19%) from the HC group. We found differences between extreme IgG levels in MDD versus HC groups and in IBS versus HC groups. Patients with MDD had significantly higher serum levels of total IgG antibodies and IgG against celery, garlic and gluten compared with healthy controls. The MDD group also had higher serum IgG levels against gluten compared with the IBS group. Our results suggest dissimilarity in immune responses against food proteins between the examined groups, with the highest immunoreactivity in the MDD group. Further studies are needed to repeat and confirm these results in bigger cohorts and also examine clinical utility of IgG-based elimination diet in patients with MDD and IBS.

Keywords: major depressive disorder; irritable bowel syndrome; immunoglobulin G antibody; food antigen; low-grade inflammation; gut-brain axis; food hypersensitivity; food allergy; intestinal permeability

1. Introduction

Depression is an etiologically and clinically heterogeneous psychiatric disorder [1] which affects more than 300 million people worldwide [2]. Its development is connected with both genetic determinants and environmental factors [3,4]. In 1991, Smith formulated the macrophage theory of depression which suggested that mechanisms involved in the pathogenesis of the disease are macrophage activation and excessive secretion of pro-inflammatory cytokines. Pro-inflammatory cytokines, due to their ability to penetrate the blood–brain barrier (BBB), may influence the metabolism and secretion of neurotransmitters which, consequently, leads to dysregulation of Central Nervous System (CNS) homeostasis [5]. There is a vast body of evidence in support of this theory: (1) the imbalance of pro-inflammatory and anti-inflammatory mediators is observed before the onset of the illness [6]; (2) significantly higher levels of pro-inflammatory cytokines are observed in the acute phase of depression [7]; (3) higher levels of inflammation markers are linked to a higher risk of recurrence of the next depressive episode [8]; (4) higher concentrations of markers of inflammation are connected with progression of the illness [9]; (5) a wide range of anti-inflammatory agents have been successfully tested in patients suffering from major depressive disorder (MDD) [10].

Factors related to systemic inflammation include i.a. excessive stress, environmental pollution, stimulants (cigarettes, alcohol), excessive body weight, poor diet [11] and leaky gut syndrome [12,13]. An increasing number of studies show a probable relationship between systemic inflammation and gut permeability in such conditions as: coeliac disease [14], autoimmune hepatitis [15], Parkinson's disease [16], autism spectrum disorders [17,18]. In 2017, Karakula-Juchnowicz et al. suggested that IgG food hypersensitivity could lead to systemic inflammation and be a trigger factor for the development of MDD. Proteins that occur in food and protein-derived compounds may modulate the immune response of the body. Increased gut permeability may lead to translocation of food-borne components into blood circulation, resulting in an abnormal immune response and increased levels of circulating pro-inflammatory cytokines, and thus, the development or maintenance of MDD. Elimination of trigger foods may inhibit the pathological response of the immune system and restore the pro/anti-inflammatory balance of the body [19] (see Figure 1 for an overview).

There is growing evidence that one of the most visible manifestations of gut permeability is irritable bowel syndrome (IBS) which affects 10–13% people around the world [20]. What is more, it is documented that individuals with IBS present low-grade intestinal inflammatory process [21], which is not always connected with a history of a gastrointestinal infection [22]. Irritable bowel syndrome, the most common group of gastrointestinal symptoms characterized by diarrhoea, constipation and bloating, can affect quality of life in those patients [23]. Abdominal pain or discomfort associated with IBS is relieved by defecation. Subtypes of IBS are distinguished based on the manifested symptoms: IBS with constipation (IBS-C), IBS with diarrhoea (IBS-D), mixed IBS (IBS-M), unsubtyped IBS [24].

The etiology of IBS has not been fully elucidated. However, some determinants known as gut-permeability-inducers (e.g., microbiota alternation and diet), have been suggested to play a role in pathophysiology of IBS [25]. Due to the characteristics of IBS (no organic changes), the treatment is based on changes of lifestyle, dietary interventions, counselling, psychological therapies, and dealing with symptoms [26]. Pharmacological therapies that target IBS symptoms include: antispasmodic medication with laxative or anti-diarrhoeal therapies; antibiotics, probiotics, bulking agents, stool softeners or stimulant laxatives [27,28]. Elimination diets are key to reducing IBS symptoms like bloating, gas and pain. The most recommended one is a low FODMAP diet (eliminating fermentable oligosaccharides, disaccharides, monosaccharides and polyols) [29,30] which is followed by a gluten-free diet according to non-celiac gluten sensitivity (NCGS) [31,32], a lactose-free diet [33] or a diet based on measurements of individual levels of IgG antibodies to food antigens in patients [34]. The efficacy of a low FODMAP diet is around 75% in patients with visceral hypersensitivity [35], but on the other hand, a low FODMAP diet might alter gut microbiota. FODMAPs belong to foods that have prebiotic functions, therefore their restriction may lead to reduction in beneficial bacteria in faeces (*Bifidobacteria*) [36].

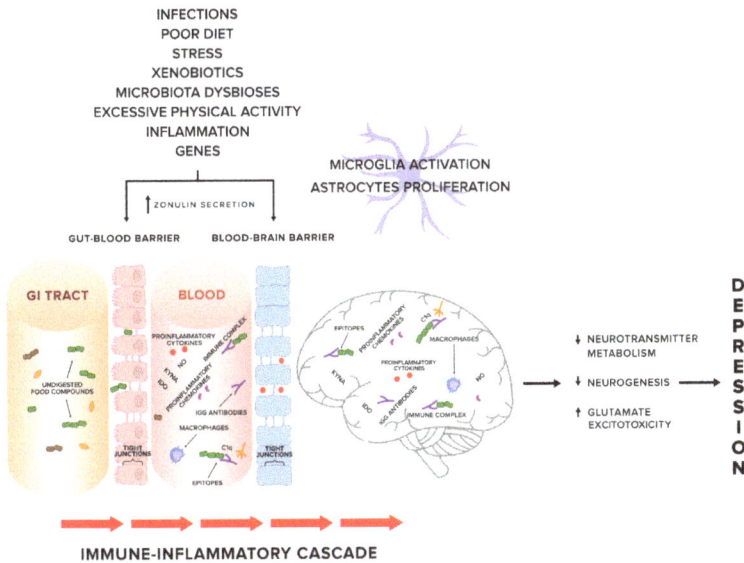

Figure 1. The gut-immune-inflammatory-brain model for Major Depressive Disorder associated with food IgG hyperreactivity. According to the hypothesis proposed in our previous work [19], we present a possible mechanism underlying the MDD development, suggesting that the interplay between genetic and environmental factors may lead to disruption of tight junctions, the loss of their integrity and both gut and BBB permeability. Undigested food compounds, which would normally break down in the gut, translocate into the blood circulation, and trough epitopes combine with food IgG antibodies to form immune complexes. This, in turn, provokes an abnormal response and triggers immune-inflammatory cascade. Uncontrolled release of the proinflammatory mediators may contribute to low-grade systemic inflammation and low-grade neuroinflammation, which, via pathological processes in CNS, i.e., changes in neurotransmitter metabolism, neurogenesis, glutamate excitotoxicity, may in consequence induce and then maintain and prolong depression. Abbreviations: GI tract, gastrointestinal tract; KYNA, kynurenic acid; NO, nitrogen oxide; IDO, indoleamine 2,3-dioxygenase; C1q, complement component 1q.

An elimination diet based on specific IgG antibodies against food has been shown to improve symptoms in patients with IBS [27,37,38]. In 2006, Monsbakken suggested that food hyperreactivity can affect up to 70% of IBS patients [39] and the number of studies confirming this finding is still growing [40,41].

Given that there is:

(1) increasing evidence linking IBS and food IgG hyperreactivity, and
(2) a suggested relationship between food IgG reactivity and MDD.

We decided to compare IgG reactions to food proteins in the serum of patients with IBS, MDD and healthy controls.

2. Material and Methods

2.1. Participants

Sixty five subjects aged 18–60 years participated in the study, including: 22 outpatients with a *DSM-5* diagnosis of major depressive disorder (MDD) [42], 22 outpatients who met Rome III Criteria [24] for the diagnosis of irritable bowel syndrome (IBS) and 21 healthy controls (HC) with no current or past history of IBS or psychiatric disorders. The mean age and sex ratio were matched across the three groups.

Exclusion criteria were as follows: (1) Body Mass Index (BMI) below 18.5 kg/m² or above 30 kg/m² (due to the possibility of either excessive or insufficient exposure to antigens, abnormal gut permeability [43–45] and changes in the gut microbiota among underweight and overweight subjects [45–47]); (2) prior or current medical history of organic brain dysfunctions; (3) a lifetime IBS diagnosis in the MDD group; (4) a lifetime MDD diagnosis in the IBS group (5) meeting criteria for substance abuse/dependence or mental retardation; (6) current use of anti-inflammatory or anti-allergic medications or antibiotics; (7) any inflammatory, oncological or systemic immune disease, diabetes mellitus, infectious diseases; (8) following any types of specific diets; (9) pregnancy or lactation.

The study was conducted in accordance with the Declaration of Helsinki, and the protocol was approved by the Ethics Committee of Medical University of Lublin (the project identification code: KE-0254/127/2016). After description of the study, a written informed consent was obtained from every subject.

2.2. Concentration of Specific IgG Antibodies

The fasting sera were examined for the concentration of specific IgG against 39 selected foods using enzyme-linked immunosorbent assay (ELISA), according to the manufacturer's recommendations (ImuPro test; R-Biopharm, Darmstadt, Germany), which was described previously [48]. Standardized calibration curve for IgG was performed according to 1st WHO IRP 67/86 for human IgG. Quantitative measurements are shown in µg/mL. All values above 7.5 µg/mL were considered as a positive reaction to a certain food. The full list of food antigens tested includes: vegetables (broccoli, carrot, cucumber, sweet pepper, red cabbage, tomato, celery, soya beans); fruits (pineapple, watermelon, cherry); spices (horseradish, garlic, mustard seed); meat (pork, beef, chicken); eggs (chicken egg); cereals with gluten (gluten, barley, oat, wheat, spelt, rye); seeds and nuts (poppy seed, almond, hazelnut, peanut, pistachio, linseed, sunflower seed); fish & seafood (crayfish); milk products (cow's: milk, sour-milk products, rennet cheese, goat's: milk and cheese, sheep's: milk and cheese); sugar products (honey) and yeast (bakery yeast).

2.3. Statistical Analysis

Earlier studies demonstrated the skewed distributions of data on IgG antibodies concentrations [49]. In view of the possibility of weakness of results obtained from classical statistical analysis and changes the reliability of analysis after a log-transformation we decided to use the ex-Gaussian statistics which is more advanced and could detect an important dissimilarity in groups with extreme results of IgG plasma levels.

The ex-Gaussian modelling of raw biological data was conducted to illustrate the specificity of quantitative results in a way that best reflects the distribution of the parameters studied. The ex-Gaussian statistics were used to compare the unprocessed results we obtained for the groups, without the need to remove the selected results or to convert the results artificially in order to adjust them to Gaussian distribution, but to take into account their exponential specificity.

The use of the ex-Gaussian statistics makes it possible to estimate three independent parameters: mu (μ) representing the mean of the normal component, reflecting the average IgG results in each group, sigma (σ) corresponding to the symmetrical standard deviation of the normal component, showing the variability of raw results, and tau (τ), containing the exponential part of the distribution, displaying the extremes in IgG results. Comparisons of mu and tau between three studied groups will show factual differences in two separated aspects of IgG outcomes: averaged, most frequently occurring results, and the comparison of tau will indicate which group has the highest number of individuals with clinically high IgG titers.

The modelling of ex-Gaussian parameters was performed with the MATLAB toolbox "DISTRIB". Data pre-processing allowing correct export of the results to the MATLAB software was proceeded with an individually customized Excel macro. All further operations were conducted according to Lacouture and Cousineau [50] recommendations for applying ex-Gaussian modelling to experimental data. Figure 2 confirms that the data obtained for all IgG results in all three groups match closely to the specificity of the ex-Gaussian distribution.

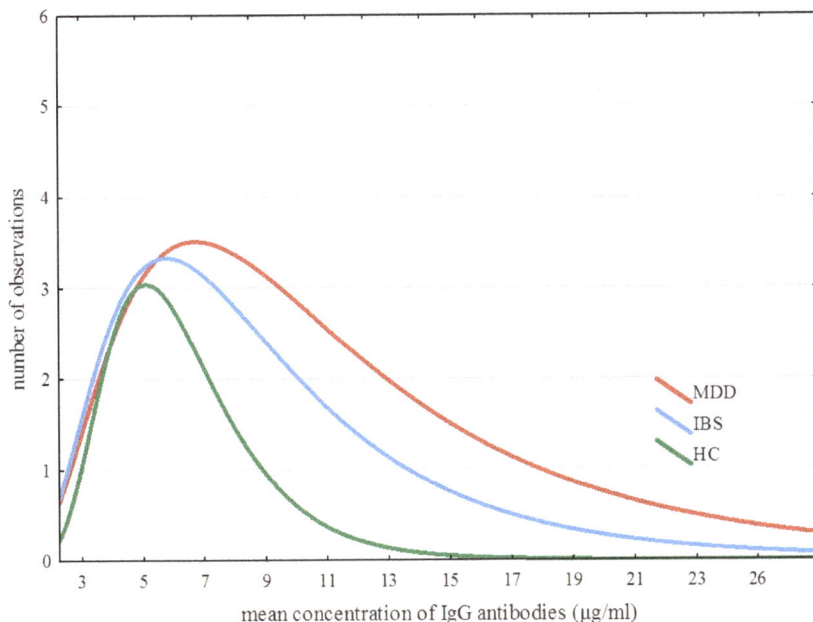

Figure 2. Specific traits of distribution of averaged results across all groups.

Due to the skewed distribution of IgG data, the comparison of obtained ex-Gaussian parameters (μ, σ and τ) for three groups was conducted with the omnibus Kruskal–Wallis rank-based nonparametric H test for comparison of more than two groups. In the case of results confirming the significant between-group difference, *post-hoc* analysis was performed with the median test, an extension of Kruskal–Wallis test enabling the comparison of all groups in pairs. This solution has been chosen instead of Mann–Whitney statistics as a *post-hoc* test, because the ranks that the pair-wise Mann–Whitney test use are not the ranks used by the Kruskal–Wallis test. Relinquishing of the Mann-Whitney test as a *post-hoc* analysis method will also reduce the risk of type I error occurrence [51].

The further statistical exploration was focused on establishing the between-group differences regarding the individual IgG results. This step of the statistical analysis was dependent on the result of the comparison concerning the ex-Gaussian parameters. When the comparison showed a significant difference between two groups, the Mann–Whitney test was used. When the difference concerned three groups, the Kruskal–Wallis test was applied, similarly as with the ex-Gaussian parameters.

All statistical analyses were performed using STATISTICA 12 (TIBCO Software Inc., CA, USA) for Windows and MATLAB software (version: R2017a, Mathworks Inc., Natick, MA, USA).

3. Results

3.1. Characteristics of the Examined Groups

General characteristics of the participants are shown in Table 1. There were no differences in age or alcohol intake between the examined groups. The MDD group had higher BMI and lower levels of physical activity compared with the IBS group. The median of coffee intake (cups/day) was higher in MDD (two cups of coffee a day) compared with IBS and HC group (0 cup of coffee a day). Interestingly, both MDD and the IBS group had more severe gastric complaints (measured during the week prior to the examination by the scale which subjectively assessed frequency and severity of symptoms; the sum of complaints ranged from 0 to 10) compared with the HC group.

Duration of illness ranged from 0.5 to 22 years across the MDD group and from 3 to 36 years across the IBS group. Three (13.63%) of the MDD patients experienced their first episode of depression, 18 (86.37%) patients had a recurrent episode of depression (the number of episodes ranging from two to 11 episodes). Eleven (50%) from MDD patients received selective serotonin reuptake inhibitors (SSRIs), four (18.18%) patients were taking Venlafaxine, five (22.73%) patients were treated with Trazodone and two (9.09%) with Mianserine. Six (31.82%) from the IBS patients had IBS with constipation, four (18.18%) IBS with diarrhoea, five (22.73%) mixed IBS and three (13.64%) unspecific IBS.

Twenty-nine (44.62%) of the patients reported using a diet in the past. Five (7.70%) patients had tried a diet with caloric restriction, including two (9.09%), two (9.09%) and one (4.76%) participants from MDD, IBS and HC group, respectively. Among sixteen (24.62%) patients who had been following an elimination diet, there had been six (27.27%) patients from the MDD group, six (27.27%) from the IBS group and four (19.05%) from HC group (see Supplementary Materials Table S1). At the moment of the examination, none of the patients were on a diet, which was one of the exclusion criteria.

Table 1. Characteristic of studied groups.

	MDD (*n* = 22)	IBS (*n* = 22)	HC (*n* = 21)	Analysis	Post-hoc Analysis
Age	31.5 (14.5)	38.5 (15.3)	34 (25)	H = 1.36, *p* = 0.506	–
Gender (% male)	50	45.4	57.1	χ^2 = 1.17, *p* = 0.554	–
BMI	28.6 (3.2)	22.8 (5.5)	25.8 (5.9)	H = 9.59, *p* = 0.005	MDD > IBS
Physical activity *	1 (0)	2 (0.3)	2 (1.5)	H = 7.77, *p* = 0.021	MDD < IBS
Number of cigarettes per day	0 (2.25)	0 (0)	0 (0)	H = 2.45, *p* = 0.294	–
Number of cups of coffee per day	2 (2)	0 (0)	0 (2)	H = 22.32, *p* <0.001	MDD > IBS MDD > HC
Intake of alcohol	4 (7.5)	4 (1)	3.5 (3.3)	H = 2.11, *p* = 0.348	–
Gastric complaints *	6.5 (6)	5 (5.5)	1 (3)	H = 16.25, *p* <0.001	MDD > HC IBS > HC
Duration of illness	5 (8)	3 (11.5)	–	Z = 0.94, *p* = 0.35	–

Values are shown as median (interquartile range); MDD—major depressive disorder; IBS—irritable bowel syndrome; HC—healthy controls; BMI—body mass index; H—H-value; *p*—*p*-value; χ^2—χ^2-value; Z—Z-value; * based on 10-point scale.

3.2. Seroreactivity to Food Antigens in the Examined Groups

IgG food hyperreactivity (interpreted as an average of levels of IgG antibodies above 7.5 µg/mL) was detected in 28 (43%) participants: 14 (64%) from the MDD group, ten (46%) from the IBS group and four (19%) from the HC group.

Due to substantially skewed data with increased exponential part of distribution, we decided to examine the differences in the ex-Gaussian parameters (which include differences of the normal component— σ and the extremes— τ) of total IgG serum levels between the three groups.

Figure 2 shows specific traits of distribution of averaged results across all three groups. Detailed analysis of ex-Gaussian distribution of total IgG values suggests a dissimilarity in immune responses between participants from the examined groups. The outliers of IgG levels are shaped from approximately 19–28, from approximately 14–20 and from approximately 9–13 in the MDD, IBS and HC groups, respectively.

As shown in Table 2, there were no significant differences in µ and σ parameters between the three groups. However, statistically significant differences were found in τ parameter between the examined groups. The *post-hoc* analysis revealed differences between MDD and HC groups and between IBS and HC groups.

Table 2. Differences in IgG normal part of data distribution (μ), symmetrical standard deviation (σ) and exponential part of IgG levels dispersion (τ).

ex-Gaussian Parameters	MDD *M*	IBS *M*	HC *M*	H (2, 65)	*p*	*Post-hoc* Analysis
μ	1.640	1.820	2.027	1.178	0.554	–
σ	0.001	0.175	0.463	0.883	0.642	–
τ	8.088	5.692	2.616	19.389	0.0001	MDD > HC IBS > HC

Post-hoc analysis: MDD–HC: major depressive disorder–healthy controls, *p* < 0.00001; IBS–HC: irritable bowel syndrome–healthy controls, *p* = 0.018; *M*—median; H—Kruskal-Wallis non-parametric ANOVA; *p*—*p*-value.

The comparison of serum IgG levels against various food proteins between the examined groups analysed by Kruskal–Wallis non-parametric ANOVA and the results after *post-hoc* test are shown in Table 3. We present only statistically significant results. A comparison of IgG antibodies against all analysed food proteins was summarized in Supplementary Materials (see Tables S2 and S3).

Table 3. Differences in serum IgG levels against tested food proteins.

IgG	G	M	IQR	Min	Max	Kruskal–Wallis H Test for 3 Groups		Post-hoc Analysis	
						H	p	Groups	p
Total IgG	MDD	403.9	365.1	109.68	1075.11	7.90	0.019	MDD > HC	0.004
	IBS	308.6	282.1	108.07	1041.08				
	HC	219.3	70.2	130.20	657.15				
Broccoli	MDD	5.29	3.16	1.52	21.85	6.20	0.045	MDD > HC	0.039
	IBS	4.73	2.72	1.79	10.43				
	HC	3.56	1.04	1.62	6.40				
Celery	MDD	6.15	6.80	1.58	28.20	8.03	0.017 *	MDD > HC	0.019
	IBS	4.53	4.74	1.52	12.43				
	HC	2.87	2.14	1.14	7.32				
Horseradish	MDD	4.08	3.66	1.42	48.10	6.98	0.030	MDD > HC	0.024
	IBS	4.02	2.68	1.51	11.43				
	HC	2.77	0.89	1.08	6.79				
Garlic	MDD	6.33	7.02	1.01	75.64	7.88	0.017 *	MDD > HC	0.015
	IBS	2.92	4.98	0.75	15.83				
	HC	2.49	1.19	0.95	10.77				
Gluten	MDD	16.44	16.10	5.26	112.61	10.37	0.005 *	MDD > HC	0.025
	IBS	8.87	10.43	2.26	117.87			MDD > IBS	0.010
	HC	11.74	7.40	3.94	43.01				
Wheat	MDD	15.26	16.38	4.56	99.42	6.79	0.033	MDD > HC	0.043
	IBS	9.31	8.05	2.28	122.13				
	HC	8.60	5.53	3.28	47.22				
Rye	MDD	11.41	8.42	3.73	108.92	7.23	0.026	MDD > HC	0.032
	IBS	7.38	8.14	2.10	28.52				
	HC	5.59	4.94	2.08	38.05				
Sunflower seed	MDD	6.22	5.84	1.43	46.15	7.07	0.029	MDD > IBS	0.038
	IBS	3.06	2.94	0.91	68.05				
	HC	3.13	2.45	0.74	61.62				
Milk products	MDD	27.57	39.82	1.62	110.57	7.59	0.025	MDD > HC	0.019
	IBS	20.00	42.78	1.24	119.30				
	HC	6.86	5.46	0.96	86.24				

* Differences statistically significant also after *post-hoc* analysis; G—group; *M*—median; IQR—interquartile range; H—H-value; *p*—*p*-value. MDD—major depressive disorder; IBS—irritable bowel syndrome; HC—healthy controls.

There was a difference in total serum IgG levels between MDD and HC groups. Patients suffering from MDD had significantly higher serum levels of total examined IgG antibodies. An analysis of individual IgG levels revealed that patients with MDD had significantly higher IgG levels against broccoli, celery, horseradish, garlic, gluten, wheat, rye and milk products compared with HC group. The MDD group also had statistically higher serum IgG levels against gluten and sunflower seed compared with IBS patients. After *post-hoc* analysis, statistical significance was achieved only by results in differences of serum concentrations of IgG against celery, garlic and gluten between MDD and HC groups and against gluten between MDD and the IBS groups.

We find no correlations between gender, age, BMI, number of cigarettes and cups of coffee per day, intake of alcohol, physical activity, duration of illness and serum total IgG levels across the examined groups. Similarly, correlations between gastric complaints and serum IgG levels were not found in IBS and HC groups. However, there was a positive correlation between total IgG level and gastric complaints in the MDD group ($p < 0.05$; $R = 0.66$).

We performed another statistical analysis on the group of IBS patients divided into two subgroups, i.e., with diarrhoea (IBS-D) and non-diarrhoea (IBS-ND). We did not find any differences either in the total IgG levels ($p > 0.05$) or in the levels of specific IgG antibodies ($p > 0.05$) between the IBS-D and IBS-ND patients. Focusing on differences between IBS subtypes seems to be a promising avenue for future research on bigger groups of patients suffering from IBS. As for our study, due to unequal numbers of patients in 4 groups resulting from the division of the IBS group, multiple-group analysis could not be conducted.

4. Discussion

There are numerous studies which confirm IgG hyperreactivity to food antigens in patients with IBS [27,38,52–59].

Due to this substantial amount of evidence and an unclear association between MDD and IgG hyperreactivity, we decided to compare levels of IgG antibodies against food between IBS, MDD patients and healthy controls.

The results of our study indicate differences between the examined groups in the proportion of people whose total IgG values exceeded the cut off level (>7.5 µg/mL). Unusually, most cases of hyperreactivity were found in MDD (64%) group and the least number in HC (19%) group. As revealed by the *post-hoc* comparisons of the paired groups, total IgG in the examined groups showed differences between MDD patients and healthy controls, no such dissimilarity was found between the IBS group and HC group. It was the application of ex-Gaussian modelling (due to substantially skewed data with increased exponential part of distribution) that revealed differences in tau (τ) (which displays the extremes in IgG results) between MDD and HC groups and also between the IBS and HC groups.

Further analysis demonstrated the presence of many distinctions in individual levels of IgG depending on the type of illness. There were differences in levels of IgG against celery, garlic and gluten between MDD and HC groups and levels of IgG against gluten between the IBS and MDD groups.

Our results indicate a dissimilarity in the immune response to food antigens among the three studied groups, surprisingly, with the highest immunoreactivity in patients suffering from MDD compared with healthy controls. A possible mechanism of the phenomenon remains obscure.

On the one hand, a possible cause of the hyperreactivity among patients with MDD may be disruption of gut-microbiome-brain axis, which is related to low-grade inflammation occurring peripherally and in the CNS [19]. It is suggested that altered gut microbiota could be responsible for increased gut permeability.

Evidence from model studies confirms that intragastric administration of *Clostridium butyricum* contributes to improvements in mucosa and BBB integrity and inhibition of neuroinflammation processes [60]. What is more, one recent study on patients with mood disorders revealed that the disruption of gut barrier integrity could be a result of gut dysbiosis. Based on the analysis of fecal microbiota, researchers demonstrated that patients with MDD and anxiety were characterized by over-representation of genes involved in LPS biosynthesis and deleterious metabolism of mood neurotransmitter pathways. The patients with mood disorders had also higher levels of plasma LPS, zonulin and fatty-acid binding protein 2 (FABP2) which reflected gut permeability [61]. However, it is still poorly understood whether intestinal barrier dysfunction is a cause or a consequence of MDD or it exists merely in some group of patients regardless of the disease.

On the other hand, there is some evidence that due to gut-brain signaling, inflammation of CNS could lead to secondary disruptions of the digestive tract. More and more studies show that neuroinflammation is a cause of chronic mucosal damage in the gut and hyperreactivity of enteric glial cells. The intestinal barrier disruptions manifest themselves by long-term neurobehavioral changes [62,63]. Post-mortem studies demonstrated that neuroinflammation was involved in pathophysiology of depression [64,65].

A scenario proposed by Karakula-Juchnowicz et al. that links the inflammatory theory of depression with IgG food hypersensitivity and leaky gut syndrome assumes that loss of integrity of the tight-junction barrier could be caused by food antigens [19]. Overproduction of zonulin triggered, for example, by gliadin through activation of the epidermal growth factor receptor and protease-activated receptor causes loosening of the tight junction barrier and an increase in permeability of the gut wall. Afterwards, intestinal permeability allows food-derived compounds cross into bloodstream and activate the immune response which is involved in overproduction of proinflammatory cytokines, their transport across BBB and, consequently, the presence of clinical manifestation of depression [19]. There is a substantial body of evidence that there is a link between food-derived antigens and other psychiatric disorders with the suggested role of inflammation in their pathogenesis [66]. Okusaga et al. revealed a possible relationship between non-celiac gluten sensitivity dependent on IgG antibodies and inflammatory pathways. In the mentioned study, schizophrenic patients with elevated anti-gliadin IgG had increased serum kynurenine levels and kynurenine to tryptophan ratio compared with patients without increased anti-gliadin IgG. Tryptophan to kynurenine conversion is linked with inflammation and raised cortisol levels [67]. Another study found that anti-casein IgG antibodies are linked with type I bipolar disorder, psychotic symptoms and mania severity [68].

So far, the number of studies exploring seroreactivity to food antigens in patients with MDD has been insufficient. Only one observation has been made and its results remain inconclusive. The paper in question reports no differences in mean IgG concentrations between MDD patients and healthy persons. The researchers observed lower levels of IgG against dietary proteins in patients with MDD who had high exposure to milk proteins compared with the control group with high exposure. Surprisingly, the authors found lower levels of tumour necrosis factor-alpha (TNF-alpha) and higher levels of cortisol in sera of the patients relative to the control subjects [69]. TNF-alpha and interleukin 6 (IL-6) are considered to be well-known inflammatory factors involved in pathophysiology of depression, as supported by a meta-analysis done by Köhler et al. in 2017 [70]. Also, the results of the studies on anti-inflammatory effects of cortisol [71] have not been confirmed in MDD patients where excess cortisol secretion was associated with higher levels of proinflammatory cytokines [72]. These findings confirmed the notion that glucocorticoid resistance, cortisol hypersecretion and increased inflammation are indeed coexistent and related biological abnormalities [73]. An interesting observation made by Rudzki et al. [69] is the link between TNF-alpha concentration and total food IgG level, indicating a potential relationship between IgG reactivity to dietary proteins and low-grade inflammation. Some explanation for the discrepant results obtained by Rudzki et al. [69] may be provided by findings from the study by Lamers at al. [74] pointing to a differential role of HPA-axis function, inflammation and metabolic syndrome in melancholic versus atypical depression. The proportion of 50% of patients with melancholic depression versus 11.76% of patients with atypical depression in the study by Rudzki et al. [69] could have had a substantial influence on a lack of differences in IgG levels between the patients and the healthy controls. A relatively small size of the group of patients and statistical analysis conducted by means of classical methods may also have affected the validity of the observations.

Our results regarding differences between IBS and HC are partly consistent with findings from other studies and indicated that serum IgG antibody levels of some common foods are abnormally elevated in IBS patients [75,76]. We did not find differences in total IgG levels between IBS and HC groups until we applied ex-Gaussian modelling which allowed us find differences in the extreme results (τ) of IgG levels between these two groups. Based on elevated IgG above the cut-off point we detected dissimilarity between IBS (46%) and HC (19%). However, we did not find differences in individual levels of IgG.

This lack of consistency with findings from other studies could be a consequence of a relatively small size of the group. On the other hand, this may be explained by attempts of IBS patients to cut down on foods aggravating their symptoms such as bloating or constipation. Taking into account that gastrointestinal complaints are the core of IBS [77], patients suffering from this disorder might intuitively cut down on the food products that, in their opinion, worsen the symptoms [39,78], yet without calling this practice "following a diet". From a clinical perspective, such behaviour is not tantamount to an elimination diet, which was an exclusion criterion from our study. However, it might lead to decreased exposure to a specific food antigen, possibly affecting IgG levels. For this reason, further research aimed at finding differences in food IgG levels between the groups studied should determine food intake and eating frequency in order to evaluate exposure to the food products studied. It is worth mentioning that an elimination diet is a method used to reduce IgG antibodies in the case of high concentrations of IgG against food proteins [78]. On the other hand, results of studies concentrated on the relationship between food-IgG exposure and dietary habits are contradictory [69,79], so research aimed at assessing differences in IgG antibodies against food, especially food with high FODMAP concentration levels (e.g., garlic, gluten, broccoli), between healthy controls and IBS patients should strictly determine the time between the discontinuation of the diet and IgG examination.

A positive response to a diet based on IgG antibodies against food has been reported in several different diseases, such as migraine [49,80], obesity [81], Crohn disease [82]. A common thread of all above cases is inflammation. Recent data provide evidence that inflammatory processes are considered to be an important factor for the development of both depression and IBS [12,83,84]. To our knowledge, there are no randomized control trials supporting potential utility of an elimination diet in patients with MDD, however, it has been shown that an elimination diet based on specific IgG antibodies against food may alleviate symptoms in patients suffering from IBS [27,37–39].

In a double blind, randomized, controlled, parallel study, Atkinson et al. [27] showed significant reduction in severity of symptoms in patients with IBS due to an elimination diet based on a IgG test compared to a sham diet (not based on increased quantities of IgG-antibodies). The quality of life also improved after following an IgG-based diet. The authors calculated that three patients out of four should be treated with this approach. After reintroduction of the respective foods the researchers observed the reverse response in the patients. Those findings are consistent with a study by Drisko et al. [38]. They also show a significant improvement of symptoms in patients with IBS. The researchers demonstrated increased titres of specific IgG antibodies for selected food in this group of patients. After 6 months on a diet without products with increased IgG concentration, patients with IBS demonstrated improvement in stool frequency, pain relief and the quality of life.

In turn, Zuo et al. [52] analysed patients with IBS and FD (functional dyspepsia) in comparison to the control group in terms of specific IgG, IgE antibody and total IgE antibody titres. They demonstrated that IBS patients had significantly higher titres of IgG antibody to crab, egg, shrimp, soybean and wheat than controls. FD patients had significantly higher titres of IgG antibody to egg and soybean than controls. Interestingly, there was no correlation in percent of patients with positive specific IgE antibodies in the three groups. There were no significant differences between IBS patients, FD patients and controls in the serum total IgE antibody levels. Guo et al. [57] evaluated the benefit of an IgG-based diet in patients with IBS with diarrhoea form (IBS-D) of the disease. The phase of 12-week elimination of food products with increased IgG resulted in improvement in IBS-D participants compared with the baseline. The researchers showed amelioration in abdominal pain (bloating level and frequency), diarrhoea frequency, abdominal distension, stool shape, general feelings of distress and total symptom score.

An interesting study was conducted by Aydinlar et al. [56]. In this double-blind, randomized, controlled, cross-over clinical trial individuals suffering from both migraine and IBS could take advantage of IgG-based elimination diet. An individual diet approach may effectively alleviate conditions such as migraine attack, maximum attack duration, mean attack duration, maximum attack severity and number of attacks with acute medication, as well as abdominal symptoms: pain-bloating severity, pain-bloating within the last 10 days, and also improvement in quality of life. Nonetheless, the small sample (21 patients) and funding bias of the examination should be pointed out as a weakness of the study.

Despite many results confirming the clinical manifestation of elevated levels of IgG antibodies against food antigens, the diagnosis based on their elimination is controversial. Numerous allergy societies question the usefulness of IgG antibodies tests as a diagnostic method for assessing adverse reactions to food intake [85–88], nevertheless, some recommend using IgG antibodies tests for research purposes [88]. It is known that IgG4 is an antibody involved in the desensitization of type I allergies (IgE-dependent) [89]. There is some new evidence that patients with IBS my present increased IgG4 titres [76], but this still needs clarification. It is worth mentioning that not all subclasses of IgG are involved in desensitization. Furthermore, they are able to form an immune complex with bounded food antigens. Such complexes are destroyed by pathogenic cells which leads to the release of proinflammatory cytokines. Aljada et al. showed that food intake is able to induce significant inflammatory changes, which has been characterized by a decrease in IkappaBalpha and an increase in NF-kappaB binding, plasma C-reactive protein (CRP), and the expression of IKKalpha, IKKbeta as well as p47 (phox) subunit [90]. This state induces a low-grade inflammation condition which may be aggravating for the body. It is documented that individuals with IBS may present low-grade inflammatory process in the gut mucosa which is not always connected with a history of a gastrointestinal infection [22]. Therefore, testing IgG against food could be one of the novel diagnostic approach to identify triggers leading to inflammation in these conditions, and administration of diet based on concentration of specific IgG may exert a beneficial effect in patients with IBS and depression.

5. Conclusions

Multiple lines of evidence increasingly point towards a role of environmental factors and disrupted gut–brain axis function both in many neuropsychiatric disorders, including depression, and in gastrointestinal disorders, including IBS [19,91–93]. The wide range of factors involved in the disturbances are considered, including changes in the mucosal immune system, the microbiota dysbioses and amounts of short chain fatty acids dependent on microbiota, exposure to xenobiotics, gut permeability, food IgG antibodies [91–95].

Our findings suggest more common food-specific serum IgG hyperreactivity among patients with IBS and MDD compared with HC, which may be one of the mechanisms leading to the development of immune activation and low-grade inflammation observed in these disorders.

Interestingly, the highest reactivity was observed in the group of MDD patients, the fact that may be of great importance for both theoretical considerations on MDD etiopathogenesis and therapeutic implications for this disorder. There is no causal relationship which could confirm clinical utility of an elimination diet in patients with MDD, however, some evidence suggests reduction of symptoms in patients with IBS who followed an IgG-based elimination diet.

To the best of our knowledge, this is the first paper published worldwide to compare IgG reactivity to food antigens in patients with these two disorders and we are of the opinion that further studies are needed to repeat and confirm these results in bigger cohorts and to examine clinical utility and duration of IgG-based elimination diet in patients with MDD and with IBS.

Supplementary Materials: The following are available online at http://www.mdpi.com/2072-6643/10/5/548/s1. Table S1: Types of diets followed by participants in the past. Table S2: Differences in serum IgG levels against tested food proteins, Table S3: Frequency of elevated IgG levels in examined groups.

Author Contributions: H.K-J., M.G. and D.J. conceived and designed the experiments; H.K-J., M.G., D.J., A.B. and Z.L. performed the experiments; P.K., J.R., K.J., J.M-T. K.S-Z., and T.K. analyzed the data; M.G., K.J. contributed reagents and analysis tools. Writing of the manuscript was done by H.K-J, J.R., A.B., D.J. and Z.L. with final content reviewed by H.K-J. All authors have given approval of the final manuscript.

Acknowledgments: The authors would like to thank Ewa Wisniewska-Ligeza for excellent language and technical assistance. This study was supported by a research grant from the Medical University of Lublin (DS 192/18).

Conflicts of Interest: The authors declare no conflict of interest.

References

1. Klein, D.N.; Hajcak, G. Heterogeneity of Depression: Clinical Considerations and Psychophysiological Measures. *Psychol. Inq.* **2015**, *26*, 247–252. [CrossRef]
2. World Health Organization. Depression. Available online: http://www.who.int/mediacentre/factsheets/fs369/en/ (accessed on 5 December 2017).
3. Uher, R. Gene-environment interactions in common mental disorders: An update and strategy for a genome-wide search. *Soc. Psychiatry Psychiatr. Epidemiol.* **2014**, *49*, 3–14. [CrossRef] [PubMed]
4. Dunn, E.C.; Brown, R.C.; Dai, Y.; Rosand, J.; Nugent, N.R.; Amstadter, A.B.; Smoller, J.W. Genetic determinants of depression: Recent findings and future directions. *Harv. Rev. Psychiatry* **2015**, *23*, 1. [CrossRef] [PubMed]
5. Smith, R.S. The macrophage theory of depression. *Med. Hypotheses* **1991**, *35*, 298–306. [CrossRef]
6. Dantzer, R. Role of the Kynurenine metabolism pathway in inflammation-induced depression: Preclinical approaches. In *Inflammation-Associated Depression: Evidence, Mechanisms and Implications*; Springer: Berlin, Germany, 2016; pp. 117–138.
7. Dahl, J.; Ormstad, H.; Aass, H.; Sandvik, L.; Malt, U.; Andreassen, O. Recovery from major depressive disorder episode after non-pharmacological treatment is associated with normalized cytokine levels. *Acta Psychiatr. Scand.* **2016**, *134*, 40–47. [CrossRef] [PubMed]
8. Lopresti, A.L.; Maker, G.L.; Hood, S.D.; Drummond, P.D. A review of peripheral biomarkers in major depression: The potential of inflammatory and oxidative stress biomarkers. *Prog. Neuro-Psychopharmacol. Biol. Psychiatry* **2014**, *48*, 102–111. [CrossRef] [PubMed]
9. Young, J.J.; Bruno, D.; Pomara, N. A review of the relationship between proinflammatory cytokines and major depressive disorder. *J. Affect. Disord.* **2014**, *169*, 15–20. [CrossRef] [PubMed]
10. Köhler, O.; Benros, M.E.; Nordentoft, M.; Farkouh, M.E.; Iyengar, R.L.; Mors, O.; Krogh, J. Effect of anti-inflammatory treatment on depression, depressive symptoms, and adverse effects: A systematic review and meta-analysis of randomized clinical trials. *JAMA Psychiatry* **2014**, *71*, 1381–1391. [CrossRef] [PubMed]
11. Ruiz-Núñez, B.; Pruimboom, L.; Dijck-Brouwer, D.J.; Muskiet, F.A. Lifestyle and nutritional imbalances associated with Western diseases: Causes and consequences of chronic systemic low-grade inflammation in an evolutionary context. *J. Nutr. Biochem.* **2013**, *24*, 1183–1201. [CrossRef] [PubMed]
12. Maes, M.; Kubera, M.; Leunis, J.-C. The gut-brain barrier in major depression: Intestinal mucosal dysfunction with an increased translocation of LPS from gram negative enterobacteria (leaky gut) plays a role in the inflammatory pathophysiology of depression. *Neuroendocrinol. Lett.* **2008**, *29*, 117–124. [CrossRef]
13. Thevaranjan, N.; Puchta, A.; Schulz, C.; Naidoo, A.; Szamosi, J.; Verschoor, C.P.; Loukov, D.; Schenck, L.P.; Jury, J.; Foley, K.P. Age-Associated Microbial Dysbiosis Promotes Intestinal Permeability, Systemic Inflammation, and Macrophage Dysfunction. *Cell Host Microbe* **2017**, *21*, 455–466.e454. [CrossRef] [PubMed]
14. Fasano, A. Zonulin and its regulation of intestinal barrier function: The biological door to inflammation, autoimmunity, and cancer. *Physiol. Rev.* **2011**, *91*, 151–175. [CrossRef] [PubMed]
15. Lin, R.; Zhou, L.; Zhang, J.; Wang, B. Abnormal intestinal permeability and microbiota in patients with autoimmune hepatitis. *Int. J. Clin. Exp. Pathol.* **2015**, *8*, 5153. [PubMed]
16. Clairembault, T.; Leclair-Visonneau, L.; Coron, E.; Bourreille, A.; Le Dily, S.; Vavasseur, F.; Heymann, M.-F.; Neunlist, M.; Derkinderen, P. Structural alterations of the intestinal epithelial barrier in Parkinson's disease. *Acta Neuropathol. Commun.* **2015**, *3*, 12. [CrossRef] [PubMed]
17. Szachta, P.; Bartnicka, A.; Galecka, M.; Skonieczna-Zydecka, K. Microbiota disorders and food hypersensitivity in autism spectrum disorders; what do we know? *J. Exp. Integr. Med.* **2015**, *5*, 117–120. [CrossRef]

18. Esnafoglu, E.; Cırrık, S.; Ayyıldız, S.N.; Erdil, A.; Ertürk, E.Y.; Daglı, A.; Noyan, T. Increased serum zonulin levels as an intestinal permeability marker in autistic subjects. *J. Pediatr.* **2017**, *188*, 240–244. [CrossRef] [PubMed]

19. Karakuła-Juchnowicz, H.; Szachta, P.; Opolska, A.; Morylowska-Topolska, J.; Gałęcka, M.; Juchnowicz, D.; Krukow, P.; Lasik, Z. The role of IgG hypersensitivity in the pathogenesis and therapy of depressive disorders. *Nutr. Neurosci.* **2017**, *20*, 110–118. [CrossRef] [PubMed]

20. Lovell, R.M.; Ford, A.C. Global prevalence of and risk factors for irritable bowel syndrome: A meta-analysis. *Clin. Gastroenterol. Hepatol.* **2012**, *10*, 712–721.e714. [CrossRef] [PubMed]

21. Sinagra, E.; Pompei, G.; Tomasello, G.; Cappello, F.; Morreale, G.C.; Amvrosiadis, G.; Rossi, F.; Monte, A.I.L.; Rizzo, A.G.; Raimondo, D. Inflammation in irritable bowel syndrome: Myth or new treatment target? *World J. Gastroenterol.* **2016**, *22*, 2242. [CrossRef] [PubMed]

22. Spiller, R.C. Infection, immune function, and functional gut disorders. *Clin. Gastroenterol. Hepatol.* **2004**, *2*, 445–455. [CrossRef]

23. Li, F.X.; Patten, S.B.; Hilsden, R.J.; Sutherland, L.R. Irritable bowel syndrome and health-related quality of life: A population-based study in Calgary, Alberta. *Can. J. Gastroenterol. Hepatol.* **2003**, *17*, 259–263. [CrossRef]

24. Longstreth, G.F.; Thompson, W.G.; Chey, W.D.; Houghton, L.A.; Mearin, F.; Spiller, R.C. Functional bowel disorders. *Gastroenterology* **2006**, *130*, 1480–1491. [CrossRef] [PubMed]

25. Jeffery, I.B.; O'toole, P.W.; Öhman, L.; Claesson, M.J.; Deane, J.; Quigley, E.M.; Simrén, M. An irritable bowel syndrome subtype defined by species-specific alterations in faecal microbiota. *Gut* **2012**, *61*, 997–1006. [CrossRef] [PubMed]

26. Foxx-Orenstein, A.E. New and emerging therapies for the treatment of irritable bowel syndrome: An update for gastroenterologists. *Ther. Adv. Gastroenterol.* **2016**, *9*, 354–375. [CrossRef] [PubMed]

27. Atkinson, W.; Sheldon, T.; Shaath, N.; Whorwell, P. Food elimination based on IgG antibodies in irritable bowel syndrome: A randomised controlled trial. *Gut* **2004**, *53*, 1459–1464. [CrossRef] [PubMed]

28. Shih, D.Q.; Kwan, L.Y. All roads lead to Rome: Update on Rome III criteria and new treatment options. *Gastroenterol. Rep.* **2007**, *1*, 56. [PubMed]

29. Marsh, A.; Eslick, E.M.; Eslick, G.D. Does a diet low in FODMAPs reduce symptoms associated with functional gastrointestinal disorders? A comprehensive systematic review and meta-analysis. *Eur. J. Nutr.* **2016**, *55*, 897–906. [CrossRef] [PubMed]

30. McKenzie, Y.; Bowyer, R.; Leach, H.; Gulia, P.; Horobin, J.; O'sullivan, N.; Pettitt, C.; Reeves, L.; Seamark, L.; Williams, M. British Dietetic Association systematic review and evidence-based practice guidelines for the dietary management of irritable bowel syndrome in adults (2016 update). *J. Hum. Nutr. Diet.* **2016**, *29*, 549–575. [CrossRef] [PubMed]

31. Barmeyer, C.; Schumann, M.; Meyer, T.; Zielinski, C.; Zuberbier, T.; Siegmund, B.; Schulzke, J.-D.; Daum, S.; Ullrich, R. Long-term response to gluten-free diet as evidence for non-celiac wheat sensitivity in one third of patients with diarrhea-dominant and mixed-type irritable bowel syndrome. *Int. J. Colorectal Dis.* **2017**, *32*, 29–39. [CrossRef] [PubMed]

32. Catassi, C.; Alaedini, A.; Bojarski, C.; Bonaz, B.; Bouma, G.; Carroccio, A.; Castillejo, G.; De Magistris, L.; Dieterich, W.; Di Liberto, D. The Overlapping Area of Non-Celiac Gluten Sensitivity (NCGS) and Wheat-Sensitive Irritable Bowel Syndrome (IBS): An Update. *Nutrients* **2017**, *9*, 1268. [CrossRef] [PubMed]

33. Böhmer, C.J.; Tuynman, H.A. The effect of a lactose-restricted diet in patients with a positive lactose tolerance test, earlier diagnosed as irritable bowel syndrome: A 5-year follow-up study. *Eur. J. Gastroenterol. Hepatol.* **2001**, *13*, 941–944. [CrossRef] [PubMed]

34. Defrees, D.N.; Bailey, J. Irritable Bowel Syndrome: Epidemiology, Pathophysiology, Diagnosis, and Treatment. *Prim. Care Clin. Off. Pract.* **2017**, *44*, 655–671. [CrossRef] [PubMed]

35. Halmos, E.P. When the low FODMAP diet does not work. *J. Gastroenterol. Hepatol.* **2017**, *32*, 69–72. [CrossRef] [PubMed]

36. Hill, P.; Muir, J.G.; Gibson, P.R. Controversies and Recent Developments of the Low-FODMAP Diet. *Gastroenterol. Hepatol.* **2017**, *13*, 36.

37. Zar, S.; Mincher, L.; Benson, M.J.; Kumar, D. Food-specific IgG4 antibody-guided exclusion diet improves symptoms and rectal compliance in irritable bowel syndrome. *Scand. J. Gastroenterol.* **2005**, *40*, 800–807. [CrossRef] [PubMed]

38. Drisko, J.; Bischoff, B.; Hall, M.; McCallum, R. Treating irritable bowel syndrome with a food elimination diet followed by food challenge and probiotics. *J. Am. Coll. Nutr.* **2006**, *25*, 514–522. [CrossRef] [PubMed]
39. Monsbakken, K.; Vandvik, P.; Farup, P. Perceived food intolerance in subjects with irritable bowel syndrome–etiology, prevalence and consequences. *Eur. J. Clin. Nutr.* **2006**, *60*, 667–672. [CrossRef] [PubMed]
40. Böhn, L.; Störsrud, S.; Törnblom, H.; Bengtsson, U.; Simrén, M. Self-reported food-related gastrointestinal symptoms in IBS are common and associated with more severe symptoms and reduced quality of life. *Am. J. Gastroenterol.* **2013**, *108*, 634–641.
41. Fritscher-Ravens, A.; Schuppan, D.; Ellrichmann, M.; Schoch, S.; Röcken, C.; Brasch, J.; Bethge, J.; Böttner, M.; Klose, J.; Milla, P.J. Confocal endomicroscopy shows food-associated changes in the intestinal mucosa of patients with irritable bowel syndrome. *Gastroenterology* **2014**, *147*, 1012–1020.e1014. [CrossRef] [PubMed]
42. American Psychiatric Association (APA). *Diagnostic and Statistical Manual of Mental Disorders*, 5th ed.; American Psychiatric Publishing: Arlington, VA, USA, 2013.
43. Hossain, M.I.; Nahar, B.; Hamadani, J.D.; Ahmed, T.; Roy, A.K.; Brown, K.H. Intestinal mucosal permeability of severely underweight and nonmalnourished Bangladeshi children and effects of nutritional rehabilitation. *J. Pediatr. Gastroenterol. Nutr.* **2010**, *51*, 638–644. [CrossRef] [PubMed]
44. Gummesson, A.; Carlsson, L.M.; Storlien, L.H.; Backhed, F.; Lundin, P.; Lofgren, L.; Stenlof, K.; Lam, Y.Y.; Fagerberg, B.; Carlsson, B. Intestinal permeability is associated with visceral adiposity in healthy women. *Obesity* **2011**, *19*, 2280–2282. [CrossRef] [PubMed]
45. Genton, L.; Cani, P.D.; Schrenzel, J. Alterations of gut barrier and gut microbiota in food restriction, food deprivation and protein-energy wasting. *Clin. Nutr.* **2015**, *34*, 341–349. [CrossRef] [PubMed]
46. Karakula-Juchnowicz, H.; Pankowicz, H.; Juchnowicz, D.; Valverde Piedra, J.L.; Malecka-Massalska, T. Intestinal microbiota—A key to understanding the pathophysiology of anorexia nervosa? *Psychiatr. Pol.* **2017**, *51*, 859–870. [CrossRef] [PubMed]
47. Seganfredo, F.B.; Blume, C.A.; Moehlecke, M.; Giongo, A.; Casagrande, D.S.; Spolidoro, J.V.N.; Padoin, A.V.; Schaan, B.D.; Mottin, C.C. Weight-loss interventions and gut microbiota changes in overweight and obese patients: A systematic review. *Obes. Rev.* **2017**, *18*, 832–851. [CrossRef] [PubMed]
48. Alpay, K.; Ertaş, M.; Orhan, E.K.; Üstay, D.K.; Lieners, C.; Baykan, B. Diet restriction in migraine, based on IgG against foods: A clinical double-blind, randomised, cross-over trial. *Cephalalgia* **2010**, *30*, 829–837. [CrossRef] [PubMed]
49. Zeng, Q.; Dong, S.Y.; Wu, L.X.; Li, H.; Sun, Z.J.; Li, J.B.; Jiang, H.X.; Chen, Z.H.; Wang, Q.B.; Chen, W.W. Variable food-specific IgG antibody levels in healthy and symptomatic Chinese adults. *PLoS ONE* **2013**, *8*, e53612. [CrossRef] [PubMed]
50. Lacouture, Y.; Cousineau, D. How to use MATLAB to fit the ex-Gaussian and other probability functions to a distribution of response times. *Tutor. Quant. Methods Psychol.* **2008**, *4*, 35–45. [CrossRef]
51. Field, A.; Hole, G. *How to Design and Report Experiments*; Sage: Newcastle, UK, 2002.
52. Zuo, X.; Li, Y.; Li, W.; Guo, Y.; Lu, X.; Li, J.; Desmond, P. Alterations of food antigen-specific serum immunoglobulins G and E antibodies in patients with irritable bowel syndrome and functional dyspepsia. *Clin. Exp. Allergy* **2007**, *37*, 823–830. [CrossRef] [PubMed]
53. Isolauri, E.; Rautava, S.; Kalliomäki, M. Food allergy in irritable bowel syndrome: New facts and old fallacies. *Gut* **2004**, *53*, 1391–1393. [CrossRef] [PubMed]
54. Whorwell, P.; Lea, R. Dietary treatment of the irritable bowel syndrome. *Curr. Treat. Opt. Gastroenterol.* **2004**, *7*, 307–316. [CrossRef]
55. Anthoni, S.; Savilahti, E.; Rautelin, H.; Kolho, K.-L. Milk protein IgG and IgA: The association with milk-induced gastrointestinal symptoms in adults. *World J. Gastroenterol. WJG* **2009**, *15*, 4915. [CrossRef] [PubMed]
56. Aydinlar, E.I.; Dikmen, P.Y.; Tiftikci, A.; Saruc, M.; Aksu, M.; Gunsoy, H.G.; Tozun, N. IgG-based elimination diet in migraine plus irritable bowel syndrome. *Headache J. Head Face Pain* **2013**, *53*, 514–525. [CrossRef] [PubMed]
57. Guo, H.; Jiang, T.; Wang, J.; Chang, Y.; Guo, H.; Zhang, W. The value of eliminating foods according to food-specific immunoglobulin G antibodies in irritable bowel syndrome with diarrhoea. *J. Int. Med. Res.* **2012**, *40*, 204–210. [CrossRef] [PubMed]
58. Vazquez-Roque, M.I.; Camilleri, M.; Smyrk, T.; Murray, J.A.; Marietta, E.; O'Neill, J.; Carlson, P.; Lamsam, J.; Janzow, D.; Eckert, D. A controlled trial of gluten-free diet in patients with irritable bowel syndrome-diarrhea: Effects on bowel frequency and intestinal function. *Gastroenterology* **2013**, *144*, 903–911.e903. [CrossRef] [PubMed]

59. Mansueto, P.; D'Alcamo, A.; Seidita, A.; Carroccio, A. Food allergy in irritable bowel syndrome: The case of non-celiac wheat sensitivity. *World J. Gastroenterol. WJG* **2015**, *21*, 7089. [CrossRef] [PubMed]

60. Li, H.; Sun, J.; Du, J.; Wang, F.; Fang, R.; Yu, C.; Xiong, J.; Chen, W.; Lu, Z.; Liu, J. Clostridium butyricum exerts a neuroprotective effect in a mouse model of traumatic brain injury via the gut-brain axis. *Neurogastroenterol. Motil.* **2017**. [CrossRef] [PubMed]

61. Stevens, B.R.; Goel, R.; Seungbum, K.; Richards, E.M.; Holbert, R.C.; Pepine, C.J.; Raizada, M.K. Increased human intestinal barrier permeability plasma biomarkers zonulin and FABP2 correlated with plasma LPS and altered gut microbiome in anxiety or depression. *Gut* **2017**. gutjnl-2017-314759. [CrossRef] [PubMed]

62. Katzenberger, R.J.; Ganetzky, B.; Wassarman, D.A. The gut reaction to traumatic brain injury. *Fly* **2015**, *9*, 68–74. [CrossRef] [PubMed]

63. Ma, E.L.; Smith, A.D.; Desai, N.; Cheung, L.; Hanscom, M.; Stoica, B.A.; Loane, D.J.; Shea-Donohue, T.; Faden, A.I. Bidirectional brain-gut interactions and chronic pathological changes after traumatic brain injury in mice. *Brain Behav. Immun.* **2017**, *66*, 56–69. [CrossRef] [PubMed]

64. Torres-Platas, S.G.; Cruceanu, C.; Chen, G.G.; Turecki, G.; Mechawar, N. Evidence for increased microglial priming and macrophage recruitment in the dorsal anterior cingulate white matter of depressed suicides. *Brain Behav. Immun.* **2014**, *42*, 50–59. [CrossRef] [PubMed]

65. Setiawan, E.; Wilson, A.A.; Mizrahi, R.; Rusjan, P.M.; Miler, L.; Rajkowska, G.; Suridjan, I.; Kennedy, J.L.; Rekkas, P.V.; Houle, S. Role of translocator protein density, a marker of neuroinflammation, in the brain during major depressive episodes. *JAMA Psychiatry* **2015**, *72*, 268–275. [CrossRef] [PubMed]

66. Hart, G.R. Food-specific IgG guided elimination diet; a role in mental health? *BAOJ Nutr.* **2017**, *3*, 045.

67. Okusaga, O.; Fuchs, D.; Reeves, G.; Giegling, I.; Hartmann, A.M.; Konte, B.; Friedl, M.; Groer, M.; Cook, T.B.; Stearns-Yoder, K.A. Kynurenine and Tryptophan Levels in Patients With Schizophrenia and Elevated Antigliadin Immunoglobulin G Antibodies. *Psychosom. Med.* **2016**, *78*, 931–939. [CrossRef] [PubMed]

68. Severance, E.G.; Gressitt, K.L.; Yang, S.; Stallings, C.R.; Origoni, A.E.; Vaughan, C.; Khushalani, S.; Alaedini, A.; Dickerson, F.B.; Yolken, R.H. Seroreactive marker for inflammatory bowel disease and associations with antibodies to dietary proteins in bipolar disorder. *Bipolar Disord.* **2014**, *16*, 230–240. [CrossRef] [PubMed]

69. Rudzki, L.; Pawlak, D.; Pawlak, K.; Waszkiewicz, N.; Małus, A.; Konarzewska, B.; Gałęcka, M.; Bartnicka, A.; Ostrowska, L.; Szulc, A. Immune suppression of IgG response against dairy proteins in major depression. *BMC Psychiatry* **2017**, *17*, 268. [CrossRef] [PubMed]

70. Köhler, C.; Freitas, T.; Maes, M.; Andrade, N.; Liu, C.; Fernandes, B.; Stubbs, B.; Solmi, M.; Veronese, N.; Herrmann, N. Peripheral cytokine and chemokine alterations in depression: A meta-analysis of 82 studies. *Acta Psychiatr. Scand.* **2017**, *135*, 373–387. [CrossRef] [PubMed]

71. Coutinho, A.E.; Chapman, K.E. The anti-inflammatory and immunosuppressive effects of glucocorticoids, recent developments and mechanistic insights. *Mol. Cell. Endocrinol.* **2011**, *335*, 2–13. [CrossRef] [PubMed]

72. Zunszain, P.A.; Anacker, C.; Cattaneo, A.; Carvalho, L.A.; Pariante, C.M. Glucocorticoids, cytokines and brain abnormalities in depression. *Prog. Neuro-Psychopharmacol. Biol. Psychiatry* **2011**, *35*, 722–729. [CrossRef] [PubMed]

73. Pariante, C.M. Why are depressed patients inflamed? A reflection on 20 years of research on depression, glucocorticoid resistance and inflammation. *Eur. Neuropsychopharmacol.* **2017**, *27*, 554–559. [CrossRef] [PubMed]

74. Lamers, F.; Vogelzangs, N.; Merikangas, K.; De Jonge, P.; Beekman, A.; Penninx, B. Evidence for a differential role of HPA-axis function, inflammation and metabolic syndrome in melancholic versus atypical depression. *Mol. Psychiatry* **2013**, *18*, 692–699. [CrossRef] [PubMed]

75. Cai, C.; Shen, J.; Zhao, D.; Qiao, Y.; Xu, A.; Jin, S.; Ran, Z.; Zheng, Q. Serological investigation of food specific immunoglobulin G antibodies in patients with inflammatory bowel diseases. *PLoS ONE* **2014**, *9*, e112154. [CrossRef] [PubMed]

76. Lee, H.S.; Lee, K.J. Alterations of Food-specific Serum IgG4 Titers to Common Food Antigens in Patients With Irritable Bowel Syndrome. *J. Neurogastroenterol. Motil.* **2017**, *23*, 578. [CrossRef] [PubMed]

77. Ikechi, R.; Fischer, B.D.; DeSipio, J.; Phadtare, S. *Irritable Bowel Syndrome: Clinical Manifestations, Dietary Influences, and Management*; Healthcare, Multidisciplinary Digital Publishing Institute: Basel, Switzerland, 2017; p. 21.

78. Hayes, P.; Corish, C.; Vny, E.; Quigley, E.M.M. A dietary survey of patients with irritable bowel syndrome. *J. Hum. Nutr. Dietet.* **2014**, *27*, 36–47. [CrossRef] [PubMed]
79. Ligaarden, S.C.; Lydersen, S.; Farup, P.G. IgG and IgG4 antibodies in subjects with irritable bowel syndrome: A case control study in the general population. *BMC Gastroenterol.* **2012**, *12*, 166. [CrossRef] [PubMed]
80. Rees, T.; Watson, D.; Lipscombe, S.; Speight, H.; Cousins, P.; Hardman, G.; Dowson, A.J. A prospective audit of food intolerance among migraine patients in primary care clinical practice. *Headache Care* **2005**, *2*, 105–110.
81. Wilders-Truschnig, M.; Mangge, H.; Lieners, C.; Gruber, H.-J.; Mayer, C.; März, W. IgG antibodies against food antigens are correlated with inflammation and intima media thickness in obese juveniles. *Exp. Clin. Endocrinol. Diabet.* **2008**, *116*, 241–245. [CrossRef] [PubMed]
82. Bentz, S.; Hausmann, M.; Piberger, H.; Kellermeier, S.; Paul, S.; Held, L.; Falk, W.; Obermeier, F.; Fried, M.; Schölmerich, J. Clinical relevance of IgG antibodies against food antigens in Crohn's disease: A double-blind cross-over diet intervention study. *Digestion* **2010**, *81*, 252–264. [CrossRef] [PubMed]
83. Piche, T. Tight junctions and IBS-the link between epithelial permeability, low-grade inflammation, and symptom generation? *Neurogastroenterol. Motil.* **2014**, *26*, 296–302. [CrossRef] [PubMed]
84. Sentsova, T.; Vorozhko, I.; Isakov, V.; Morozov, S.; Shakhovskaia, A. Immune status estimation algorithm in irritable bowel syndrome patients with food intolerance. *Exp. Clin. Gastroenterol.* **2014**, *7*, 13–17.
85. Stapel, S.O.; Asero, R.; Ballmer-Weber, B.; Knol, E.; Strobel, S.; Vieths, S.; Kleine-Tebbe, J. Testing for IgG4 against foods is not recommended as a diagnostic tool: EAACI Task Force Report. *Allergy* **2008**, *63*, 793–796. [CrossRef] [PubMed]
86. Carr, S.; Chan, E.; Lavine, E.; Moote, W. CSACI Position statement on the testing of food-specific IgG. *Allergy Asthma Clin. Immunol.* **2012**, *8*, 12. [CrossRef] [PubMed]
87. Sicherer, S.H.; Allen, K.; Lack, G.; Taylor, S.L.; Donovan, S.M.; Oria, M. Critical Issues in Food Allergy: A National Academies Consensus Report. *Pediatrics* **2017**, *140*, e20170194. [CrossRef] [PubMed]
88. Chabane, H.; Doyen, V.; Bienvenu, F.; Adel-Patient, K.; Vitte, J.; Mariotte, D.; Bienvenu, J. Les dosages d'IgG anti-aliments: Méthodes et pertinence clinique des résultats. Position du groupe de travail de biologie de la Société française d'allergologie. *Revue Française d'Allergologie* **2018**. Available online: https://www.sciencedirect.com/science/article/pii/S1877032018300289 (accessed on 11 April 2018). [CrossRef]
89. Engelhart, S.; Glynn, R.J.; Schur, P.H. Disease associations with isolated elevations of each of the four IgG subclasses. *Semin. Arthritis and Rheum.* **2017**, *47*, 276–280. [CrossRef] [PubMed]
90. Aljada, A.; Mohanty, P.; Ghanim, H.; Abdo, T.; Tripathy, D.; Chaudhuri, A.; Dandona, P. Increase in intranuclear nuclear factor κB and decrease in inhibitor κB in mononuclear cells after a mixed meal: Evidence for a proinflammatory effect. *Am. J. Clin. Nutr.* **2004**, *79*, 682–690. [CrossRef] [PubMed]
91. Abautret-Daly, Á.; Dempsey, E.; Parra-Blanco, A.; Medina, C.; Harkin, A. Gut-brain actions underlying comorbid anxiety and depression associated with inflammatory bowel disease. *Acta Neuropsychiatr.* **2017**, 1–22. [CrossRef] [PubMed]
92. Powell, N.; Walker, M.M.; Talley, N.J. The mucosal immune system: Master regulator of bidirectional gut-brain communications. *Nat. Rev. Gastroenterol. Hepatol.* **2017**, *14*, 143–159. [CrossRef] [PubMed]
93. Delaney, S.; Hornig, M. Environmental Exposures and Neuropsychiatric Disorders: What Role Does the Gut–Immune–Brain Axis Play? *Curr. Environ. Health Rep.* **2018**, *5*, 158–169. [CrossRef] [PubMed]
94. Rios-Covian, D.; Ruas-Madiedo, P.; Margolles, A.; Gueimonde, M.; de Los Reyes-Gavilan, C.G.; Salazar, N. Intestinal Short Chain Fatty Acids and their Link with Diet and Human Health. *Front. Microbiol.* **2016**, *7*, 185. [CrossRef] [PubMed]
95. Quigley, E.M.M. The Gut-Brain Axis and the Microbiome: Clues to Pathophysiology and Opportunities for Novel Management Strategies in Irritable Bowel Syndrome (IBS). *J. Clin. Med.* **2018**, *7*, 6. [CrossRef] [PubMed]

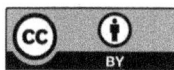

© 2018 by the authors. Licensee MDPI, Basel, Switzerland. This article is an open access article distributed under the terms and conditions of the Creative Commons Attribution (CC BY) license (http://creativecommons.org/licenses/by/4.0/).

nutrients

MDPI

Article

Dietary Sialyllactose Influences Sialic Acid Concentrations in the Prefrontal Cortex and Magnetic Resonance Imaging Measures in Corpus Callosum of Young Pigs

Austin T. Mudd [1,2], Stephen A. Fleming [1,2], Beau Labhart [3], Maciej Chichlowski [3], Brian M. Berg [3,4], Sharon M. Donovan [4,5] and Ryan N. Dilger [1,2,4,*]

[1] Piglet Nutrition & Cognition Lab, University of Illinois Urbana-Champaign, Urbana, IL 61801, USA; amudd2@illinois.edu (A.T.M.); sflemin2@illinois.edu (S.A.F.)

[2] Neuroscience Program, University of Illinois Urbana-Champaign, Urbana, IL 61801, USA

[3] Mead Johnson Pediatric Nutrition Institute, Mead Johnson Nutrition, 2400 W Lloyd Expressway, Evansville, IN 47712, USA; beau.labhart@mjn.com (B.L.); maciej.chichlowski@mjn.com (M.C.); dr.brianberg@gmail.com (B.M.B.)

[4] Division of Nutrition Sciences, University of Illinois Urbana-Champaign, Urbana, IL 61801, USA; sdonovan@illinois.edu

[5] Department of Food Science and Human Nutrition, University of Illinois Urbana-Champaign, Urbana, IL 61801, USA

* Correspondence: rdilger2@illinois.edu

Received: 1 November 2017; Accepted: 23 November 2017; Published: 28 November 2017

Abstract: Sialic acid (SA) is a key component of gangliosides and neural cell adhesion molecules important during neurodevelopment. Human milk contains SA in the form of sialyllactose (SL) an abundant oligosaccharide. To better understand the potential role of dietary SL on neurodevelopment, the effects of varying doses of dietary SL on brain SA content and neuroimaging markers of development were assessed in a newborn piglet model. Thirty-eight male pigs were provided one of four experimental diets from 2 to 32 days of age. Diets were formulated to contain: 0 mg SL/L (CON), 130 mg SL/L (LOW), 380 mg SL/L (MOD) or 760 mg SL/L (HIGH). At 32 or 33 days of age, all pigs were subjected to magnetic resonance imaging (MRI) to assess brain development. After MRI, pig serum and brains were collected and total, free and bound SA was analyzed. Results from this study indicate dietary SL influenced ($p = 0.05$) bound SA in the prefrontal cortex and the ratio of free SA to bound SA in the hippocampus ($p = 0.04$). Diffusion tensor imaging indicated treatment effects in mean ($p < 0.01$), axial ($p < 0.01$) and radial ($p = 0.01$) diffusivity in the corpus callosum. Tract-based spatial statistics (TBSS) indicated differences ($p < 0.05$) in white matter tracts and voxel-based morphometry (VBM) indicated differences ($p < 0.05$) in grey matter between LOW and MOD pigs. CONT and HIGH pigs were not included in the TBSS and VBM assessments. These findings suggest the corpus callosum, prefrontal cortex and hippocampus may be differentially sensitive to dietary SL supplementation.

Keywords: neurodevelopment; milk oligosaccharide; sialyllactose; pig; corpus callosum; sialic acid; pediatric nutrition

1. Introduction

Appropriate nutrition early in life is essential to support optimal growth and developmental trajectories in the infant. Human milk contains a unique composition of bioactive components and is generally considered the gold standard for infant nutrition [1]. While breastfeeding is ideal, it is not always a viable option, thus infant formula is often used as the sole source of nutrition for infants or in combination with some breastfeeding. Decades of research and innovation have resulted in infant formulas with a more similar composition to human milk, yet there remain compositional differences between the two [2]. Thus, ongoing research in the area of pediatric nutrition seeks to identify components of human milk that may confer physiological benefits to the neonate and may be added to the infant formula matrix. One such class of dietary components that currently differ in concentration between human milk and infant formula are oligosaccharides (OS).

As the third most abundant component of human milk, OS are thought to aid in gastrointestinal development, brain development and prevention of pathogenic events [3]. Known differences in OS concentration and composition exist between human milk and milk from other mammalian species. Notably, mature human milk contains between 3.5–14 g OS/L, whereas mature bovine milk, which is often used as a base for infant formula, contains only 0.3–0.5 g OS/L and infant formulas are reported to contain 0.4–8.0 g OS/L [4]. Additionally, 50–70% of human milk OS are fucosylated (i.e., containing a fucose molecule, neutral OS), followed by 10–30% sialylated human milk OS (i.e., containing a sialic acid (SA) molecule, acidic OS) and approximately 10% of human milk OS are neutral OS that do not contain either a fucose or SA [5].

Among the acidic OS, the most abundant human milk OS is sialyllactose (SL), which is a trisaccharide molecule composed of a SA molecule bound to lactose. Sialyllactose in milk is found predominantly in two forms, 3'-SL and 6'-SL, with the number denoting the position of the SA monosaccharide linkage to lactose [6]. Interestingly, SL has been found in many mammalian milks, including human, bovine, murine and porcine, however the concentrations of total SL and the predominant isoform of SL (i.e., either 3'-SL or 6'-SL) varies widely among species [4,7,8]. Sialyllactose contains SA which may influence neonatal brain development. Sialic acid can be obtained from the diet or produced de novo and is incorporated into glycolipid- and glycoprotein-containing molecules. Notably, SA-containing glycolipids and glycoproteins are important for synapse formation and neural transmission [9], supporting the potential importance of this molecule during a highly dynamic period of brain development. In fact, breastfed infants exhibit increased brain SA concentrations relative to formula-fed infants, further suggesting the need for SA early in life [10]. Much like the wide variation of SL concentrations in mammalian milks, brain SA concentrations appear to vary widely among species, with humans exhibiting the highest concentrations among higher order mammals [11].

Early in life, the brain is highly dynamic and thus sensitive to dietary intervention. Provided the increasing interest in milk OS and emerging evidence suggesting dietary SA may influence the brain, there exists a need to identify clinically-relevant doses at which SA-containing milk OS might support neurodevelopment. The pig is an ideal translational model for assessing the effects of nutrition on brain development, because of its similar nutritional requirements, comparable gastrointestinal development and strikingly similar brain growth trajectories [12]. Thus, the aim of this exploratory study was to elucidate the effects of varying doses of dietary SL on pig brain development using magnetic resonance imaging (MRI) and tissue SA quantification. In doing so, this study expands on current literature, which suggests the presence of SA in the diet supports early-life brain development.

2. Methods

2.1. Animal Care & Housing

Beginning at 2 days of age, 38 vaginally-derived intact male pigs were randomly assigned to one of four milk replacer diets, described below, until 32 or 33 days of age. The study was completed in 4 replicates (5–12 pigs per replicate), with pigs selected from a total of 14 litters, such that potential confounding effects of litter of origin and initial bodyweight were taken into account when allotting pigs to dietary treatments. A total of 8–11 pigs were included in each dietary treatment group. A total of 12 pigs per dietary treatment were initially started on the study, however several pigs were removed from the study for health reasons unrelated to dietary treatments. All pigs were housed in custom pig rearing units (87.6 cm length × 88.9 cm width × 50.8 cm height) fabricated with clear acrylic and stainless steel walls and vinyl-coated metal flooring. Caging units permitted pigs to see, hear, smell but not touch neighboring pigs. All pigs were provided a toy for enrichment and were allowed to physically interact with other pigs during daily cleaning (approximately 15 min per day). Pig rearing environment was maintained on a 12 h light/dark cycle, with light from 0600 to 1800 h and minimal light during the overnight dark phase. All animal care and experimental procedures were in accordance with National Research Council Guide for the Care and Use of Laboratory Animals and approved by the University of Illinois at Urbana-Champaign Institutional Animal Care and Use Committee. Approval for this research project was verified on 3 March 2015 and is identified as IACUC 15034 at the University of Illinois Urbana-Champaign.

2.2. Dietary Treatments

All diets were produced by Mead Johnson Nutrition (Evansville, IN, USA) using a proprietary blend of nutrients formulated to meet the nutritional needs of growing pigs. Pigs were provided one of 4 custom diets from 2 until 32 or 33 days of age. The control diet (CON) included docosahexaenoic acid (DHA, 87 mg/100 g milk replacer powder; DSM, Heerlen, The Netherlands), arachidonic acid (ARA, 174 mg/100 g milk replacer powder; DSM, Heerlen, The Netherlands), galactooligosaccharide (GOS, 1.0 g/100 g milk replacer powder; Friesland Campina, Zwolle, The Netherlands) and polydextrose (PDX, 1.0 g/100 g milk replacer powder; Danisco, Terre Haute, IN, USA). Experimental diets were formulated using the CON diet as the base and supplemented with bovine-derived modified whey enriched with SL (SAL-10; Arla Foods Ingredients, Aarhus, Denmark) to provide final SL concentrations of: 65 mg SL/100 g milk replacer powder (LOW), 190 mg SL/100 g milk replacer powder (MOD) and 380 mg SL/100 g milk replacer powder (HIGH). The CON diet was composed of 30% protein, 32% fat, 29% carbohydrate, 8% ash and 1% water, all test diets (i.e., LOW, MOD, HIGH) were composed of 31% protein, 32% fat, 28% carbohydrate, 8% ash and 1% water.

Milk replacer powder was reconstituted fresh each day at 200 g of dry powder per 800 g of water and pigs were fed at 285 and 325 mL of reconstituted diet per kilogram of bodyweight (BW) starting on 3 and 8 days of age, respectively. At this reconstitution rate, all diets provided equal concentrations of DHA (174 mg/L), ARA (348 mg/L) and PDX/GOS (2 g/L, each). The reconstituted experimental milk replacers were formulated to contain 130 mg SL/L (LOW), 380 mg SL/L (MOD) or 760 mg SL/L (HIGH). However, analytical assessment conducted after study completion showed the levels of SL in the diets were: 55 mg SL/L (CON), 159 mg SL/L (LOW), 429 mg SL/L (MOD) and 779 mg SL/L (HIGH) due to inherent SL in the CON diet.

2.3. Sialic Acid Quantification

For quantification of free SA, serum and tissue samples from the right hemisphere hippocampus, cerebellum and prefrontal cortex were utilized. For brain tissue, all samples were homogenized using a bead homogenization system (TissueLyser, Qiagen, Hilgden, Germany) with 3 parts of phosphate buffered saline added to 1 part of brain tissue. Serum and brain homogenate were diluted 1:10 with nanopure water, homogenized for 1 h, further diluted 1:4 with 0.10 M sodium acetate solution (brought to a pH of 5 with HCl; Fischer Scientific, Hampton, NH, USA) and filtered into an auto sampler vial for analysis. The final dilution of the free SA samples was 1:40. Acetonitrile (Sigma-Aldrich, St. Louis, MO, USA) was used in both the standards and the samples to clarify the solutions. For quantification of total SA, the samples were diluted 1:25 with nanopure water and homogenized for 1 h. Next, 250 μL of diluted sample was combined with 750 μL of enzyme solution (neuraminidase (Roche Diagnostics, Indianapolis, IN, USA) and sodium acetate buffer) and digested for 18 h in a 37 °C water bath. Post digestion, the samples were filtered directly into an auto sampler vial for analysis. The final dilution of the total SA samples was 1:100. Again, acetonitrile was used in both the standards and the samples to clarify the solutions. For analysis of both the free and total SA, samples were analyzed by ion chromatography using pulsed amperometric detection (model ICS-5000, Dionex, Sunnyvale, CA, USA). Sialic acid separation was achieved using a CarboPac PA20 column (Dionex, Sunnyvale, CA, USA) and a multi-step gradient of 0–95 mM sodium acetate in 100 mM sodium hydroxide (Fischer Scientific, Hampton, NH, USA). Sialic acid concentrations were determined via an external standard calibration curve. *N*-acetylneuramic acid (Neu5Ac standard) and *N*-glycolylneuraminic acid (Neu5Gc standard) standards were used (Sigma-Aldrich, St. Louis, MO, USA). Concentrations of free and total SA were generated from the procedures described above and concentrations of bound SA were determined by subtracting free SA from total SA concentrations, within subject. Only concentrations for Neu5Ac were above detectable limits, thus no analysis of Neu5Gc concentrations are reported herein. The ratio of free SA to bound SA was determined by dividing free SA concentrations by bound SA concentrations, within subject.

2.4. Magnetic Resonance Imaging

All pigs underwent MRI procedures on postnatal day 32 or 33 at the Beckman Institute Biomedical Imaging Center at the University of Illinois using a Siemens MAGNETOM Trio 3T scanner (Siemens Healthineers, Erlangen, Germany) with a Siemens 32-channel head coil. The pig neuroimaging protocol included three magnetization prepared rapid gradient-echo (MPRAGE) sequences and diffusion tensor imaging (DTI) to assess brain macrostructure and microstructure, respectively, as well as magnetic resonance spectroscopy (MRS) to obtain brain metabolite concentrations [13]. In preparation for MRI procedures, anesthesia was induced using an intramuscular injection of telazol (50.0 mg of tiletamine plus 50.0 mg of zolazepam reconstituted with 5.0 mL deionized water; Zoetis, Florham Park, NJ, USA) administered at 0.07 mL/kg BW and an appropriate plane of anesthesia was maintained with inhaled isoflurane (98% O_2, 2% isoflurane) delivered via a mask. Pigs were immobilized during all MRI procedures. Visual observation of each pig's well-being, as well as observations of heart rate, PO_2 and percent of isoflurane, were recorded every 5 min during the procedure and every 10 min post-procedure until animals were fully recovered. Total scan time for each pig was approximately 60 min.

2.4.1. Diffusion Tensor Imaging Acquisition and Analysis

Diffusion tensor imaging was used to assess white matter maturation and axonal tract integrity using a *b*-value = 1000 s/mm^2 across 30 directions and a 2 mm isotropic voxel. Diffusion-weighted echo-planar imaging (EPI) images were assessed using FMRIB Software Library (FSL) (FMRIB Centre, Oxford, UK) for fractional anisotropy (FA), mean diffusivity (MD), axial diffusivity (AD) and radial diffusivity (RD) using methods previously described [13]. Assessment was performed over the following regions of interest: caudate, corpus callosum, cerebellum, both hippocampi, internal capsule, left and right cortex, thalamus, DTI-generated white matter and atlas-generated white matter was performed using a customized pig analysis pipeline and the FSL software package. For the purposes of this analysis this study used the Pig Brain atlas, generated from the same species and previously reported by Conrad and colleagues [14]. The diffusion toolbox in FSL was used to generate values of AD, RD, MD and FA.

Masks for each region of interest (ROI) from the atlas were non-linearly transformed into the MPRAGE space of each individual pig and a linear transform was then applied to transfer each ROI into DTI space. A threshold of 0.5 was applied to each ROI and the data were dilated twice. For each individual ROI, an FA threshold of 0.15 was applied to ensure inclusion of only white matter in the region of interest despite the mask expansion.

2.4.2. Tract-Based Spatial Statistics

The FSL 5.0 toolbox was used for tract-based spatial statistics (TBSS) assessment of FA data. Fractional anisotropy images, previously generated from diffusion data, were manually extracted and all FA data from individual subjects were aligned using the FSL nonlinear registration tool FNIRT. Upon alignment, the study-specific mean FA image was created and a mean FA skeleton representing the center of all common tracts was established. A threshold of 0.2 was determined to be sensitive for mean FA tract delineation. Once the study-specific mean FA skeleton was created, each subjects' aligned FA data were projected onto the mean FA skeleton and the resulting voxel-wise cross-subject data were used for statistical analyses. For TBSS analysis, only pigs receiving the LOW and MOD diets were compared, thus a two-sample *t*-test was used for data analysis. Comparison between only the LOW and MOD diets was performed prior to un-blinding of dietary treatment. These treatments were specifically selected for comparison analysis based on the results of the DTI measurements. In particular, the difference between LOW and MOD in DTI analysis was the greatest of all comparisons.

The TBSS non-FA function was used to generate data on diffusion differences along the pre-determined white matter tracts for other diffusion tensor measures (i.e., MD, AD, RD). To analyze differences in these diffusion measures, nonlinear warps and skeleton projection values generated in the TBSS FA analysis were applied to each of the MD, AD and RD images. Pig-specific alterations to the non-FA script include registration to pig brain atlas space, rather than MNI152 space and registration using a pig-specific internal capsule mask rather than a lower cingulum mask. Statistical analysis for each of these diffusion measures was performed as described above for FA analysis.

2.4.3. Structural MRI Acquisition and Analysis

A T1-weighted MPRAGE sequence was used to obtain anatomic images of the pig brain, with a 0.7 isotropic voxel size. Three repetitions were acquired and averaged using SPM8 in Matlab 8.3 and brains were manually extracted using FSL (FMRIB Centre, Oxford, UK). The following sequence specific parameters were used to acquire T1-weighted MPRAGE data: repetition time (TR) = 1900 ms; echo time (TE) = 2.49 ms; 224 slices; field of view (FOV) = 180 mm; flip angle = 9°. Methods for MPRAGE averaging, manual brain extraction were previously described [13]. All data generated used a publicly-available population-averaged pig brain atlas (http://pigmri.illinois.edu) [14].

For volumetric assessments, individual brains were segmented into 19 different ROI using the pig brain atlas. Total brain and individual region volume analysis was performed in which an inverse warp file for each ROI was generated from the DARTEL-generated warp files for each region using the using the statistical parametric mapping (SPM8; Wellcome Department of Clinical Neurology, London, UK) software. Generation of region-specific warp files was previously described [15,16]. In order to account absolute whole-brain volume, all regions of interest were also expressed as a percent of total brain volume (%TBV), using the following equation: ((ROI absolute volume)/(total brain absolute volume)) × 100, within subject.

Voxel-based morphometry (VBM) analysis was performed to assess grey and white matter tissue concentrations using SPM8 software (Wellcome Department of Clinical Neurology, London, UK). Manually-extracted brains were aligned to pig brain atlas space using a 12-parameter affine transformation. The "Segment" function of SPM and pig-specific prior probability tissue maps were then used to segment the brains into grey matter and white matter. The Diffeomorphic Anatomical Registration using Exponentiated Lie Algebra (DARTEL) toolbox was used with pig-specific specifications that included changing the bounding box of −30.1 to 30.1, −35 to 44.8, −28 to 31.5; and a voxel size of 0.7 mm^3. After the nonlinear transformation of the data in the DARTEL procedure, flow fields were created and converted to warp files. The warp files generated were then applied to the subject's grey and white matter. The modulated data were smoothed with a 4 mm full-width half maximum (FWHM) and were subjected to VBM procedures using the SPM8 toolbox. For voxel-based morphometry analyses, two-sample permutation *t*-tests were performed on a voxel-by-voxel basis for grey and white matter volume differences between animals on the LOW and MOD diets, with an uncorrected $p < 0.001$. An additional threshold criterion of at least 20-edge connected voxels was used. Comparison between only the LOW and MOD diets was performed prior to un-blinding of dietary treatment. These treatments were chosen for comparison based off of the greatest difference in diffusion tensor imaging values between the treatments.

2.4.4. Magnetic Resonance Spectroscopy Acquisition and Analysis

Magnetic resonance spectroscopy was used to non-invasively quantify metabolites in the whole brain. The MRS spin-echo chemical shift sequence was used with a voxel size of 20 mm × 23 mm × 13 mm and centered over the left and right dorsal hippocampi. The following sequence parameters were used in acquisition of spectroscopy data for the water suppressed scan TR = 1800 ms; TE = 68 ms; signal averages = 256, vector size = 1024. The following sequence parameters were used in acquisition of spectroscopy data for the non-water suppressed scan TR = 20,000 ms; TE = 68 ms; signal averages = 1; vector size = 1024 point. Both water-suppressed and non-water-suppressed data were collected in institutional units and all MRS data were analyzed using LC Model (version 6.3), using methods previously described [15]. Limits were placed on MRS data for inclusion in the statistical analysis. Cramer-Rao lower bounds (i.e., % standard deviation) were calculated using the LC Model and only metabolites with standard deviation less than 20% were considered to have reliable quantitative results of absolute levels.

2.5. Statistical Analysis

All researchers involved with conducting the study and acquiring and analyzing the study results remained blinded to dietary treatment identity until final data analyses had been completed. An analysis of variance (ANOVA) was conducted using the MIXED procedure of SAS 9.4 (SAS Inst. Inc., Cary, NC, USA) to differentiate the effects of the dietary treatments provided to the pigs. All data analyzed herein were collected at a single time-point and were thus analyzed using a one-way ANOVA. No outliers (i.e., individual data-points greater than |3| studentized residuals away from the treatment mean) were detected for any measurements. The level of significance was set at $p < 0.05$ with trends accepted at $0.05 < p < 0.10$.

3. Results

3.1. Tissue & Serum Sialic Acid Quantification

For all SA quantification measures, the following number of pigs were analyzed per dietary treatment: CON ($n = 11$), LOW ($n = 9$), MOD ($n = 10$), HIGH ($n = 8$). Analysis of total and free SA indicated no differences between dietary treatments in the serum ($p = 0.67$ and 0.64, respectively), hippocampus ($p = 0.58$ and 0.23, respectively), cerebellum ($p = 0.34$ and 0.84, respectively) and prefrontal cortex ($p = 0.24$ and 0.28, respectively) (Figure 1A,B). Analysis of bound SA indicated an effect of dietary treatment ($p = 0.05$) in the prefrontal cortex. Within the prefrontal cortex, pigs on the CON diet group exhibited higher levels of bound SA compared with the LOW and MOD dietary SL groups but were not different than the HIGH dietary SL group (Figure 1C). Analysis of bound SA indicated no differences between dietary treatments in the serum ($p = 0.41$), hippocampus ($p = 0.59$), or cerebellum ($p = 0.17$). Analysis of free SA:bound SA indicated an effect of diet ($p = 0.04$) in the hippocampus, in which the MOD group exhibited a higher proportion of free SA:bound SA compared with the CON and HIGH diet groups but was not different than the LOW group (Figure 1D). Analysis of free SA:bound SA indicated no differences between dietary treatments in the serum ($p = 0.70$), cerebellum ($p = 0.18$) and prefrontal cortex ($p = 0.21$).

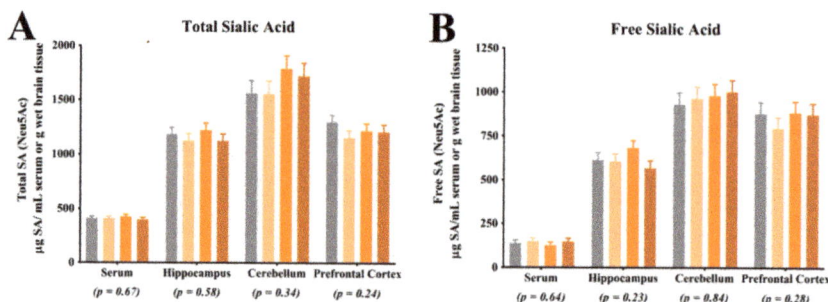

Figure 1. *Cont.*

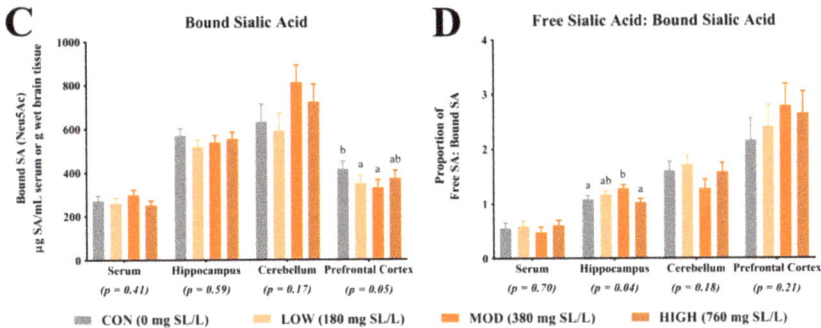

Figure 1. Bound sialic acid (SA) in the prefrontal cortex and the ratio of free SA to bound SA in the hippocampus are influenced by dietary sialyllactose (SL). (**A**) Dietary SL does not influence ($p > 0.05$) total SA in serum, hippocampus, cerebellum and prefrontal cortex; (**B**) Dietary SL does not influence ($p > 0.05$) free SA in serum, hippocampus, cerebellum and prefrontal cortex; (**C**) Dietary SL influences ($p = 0.05$) the concentration of bound SA in the prefrontal cortex; (**D**) Dietary SL influences ($p = 0.04$) the ratio of free SA to bound SA in the hippocampus. Note, serum SA concentrations are in µg/mL serum whereas brain tissue SA concentrations are in µg/g brain tissue.

3.2. Magnetic Resonance Imaging

3.2.1. Diffusion Tensor Imaging

Due to motion artifact in some of the acquired scans the following number of pigs were analyzed per dietary treatment: CON ($n = 9$), LOW ($n = 9$), MOD ($n = 7$), HIGH ($n = 7$). Diffusion tensor imaging revealed differences due to diet in corpus callosum AD ($p < 0.01$), MD ($p < 0.01$) and RD ($p = 0.01$) measures (Figure 2A). Corpus callosum MD measures were highest in the MOD group compared with CON, LOW and HIGH, which were not different from each other. Axial diffusivity measures in the corpus callosum indicated highest rates of diffusion in the MOD group when compared with all dietary treatments and HIGH pigs exhibited increased rates of diffusivity compared with LOW but not CON pigs. For RD measures, rates of diffusion were highest in MOD pigs but not different than HIGH pigs, however, rates of RD in the HIGH pigs were also not different than CON and LOW pigs. Trends for main effect of diet were observed for left hippocampus MD ($p = 0.07$) and RD ($p = 0.06$) measures, with the MOD pigs exhibiting numerically higher but not statistically significant, rates of diffusion compared with all other groups (Figure 2B). No differences due to diet were observed for MD, AD and RD measures in other analyzed ROI. Additionally, there were no differences in fractional anisotropy measures in any of the analyzed brain regions (data not shown).

3.2.2. Tract-Based Spatial Statistics

Tract-based spatial statistics (TBSS) analysis was used to identify diffusion differences between LOW diet and MOD diet pigs using study-specific, pre-determined white matter tracts. TBSS analysis of RD measures indicated a cluster of voxels in which MOD pigs exhibited higher ($p < 0.05$) RD measures when compared with LOW pigs (Figure 3, Figure S1 for full image set). Upon visual inspection, the significant voxels appear to be localized to the left hemisphere corpus callosum. The converse of this voxel-wise comparison yielded no differences in RD measures, indicating LOW pigs did not exhibit higher RD measures compared with MOD pigs, which supports DTI findings in the corpus callosum.

A

Corpus Callosum

B

Left Hippocampus

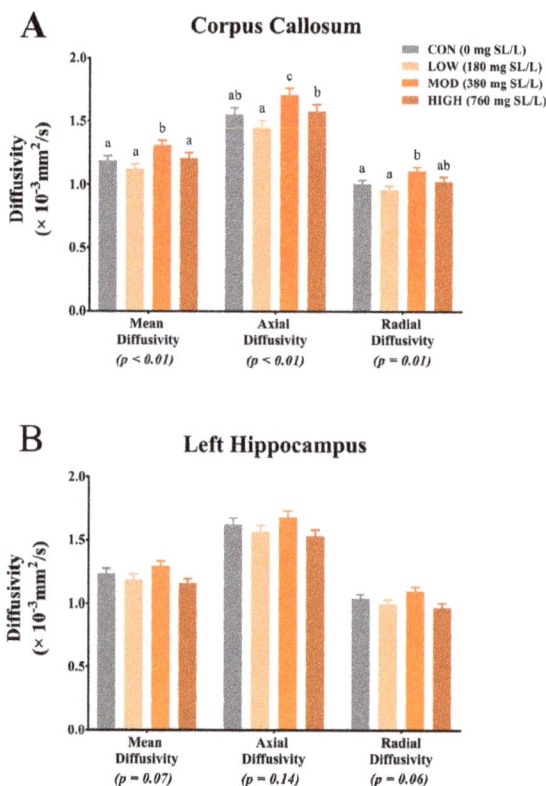

Figure 2. Diffusion tensor measures in the corpus callosum are influenced by dietary sialyllactose (SL). (**A**) Dietary SL influences diffusion tensor measures of mean diffusivity (MD) ($p < 0.01$), axial diffusivity ($p < 0.01$) and radial diffusivity (RD) ($p = 0.01$) in the corpus callosum. For all measures, pigs provided the MOD dietary SL treatment exhibited the highest rates of diffusion; (**B**) Dietary SL tended to influence ($0.05 < p < 0.10$) diffusion tensor measures of MD ($p = 0.07$) and RD ($p = 0.06$) in the left hippocampus.

Tract-based spatial statistics analyses were also performed on skeletonized masks of FA, AD and MD data. For each separate analysis, diffusion values revealed no differences ($p > 0.05$) in which pigs provided the LOW diet exhibited higher diffusion values along predetermined white matter tracts, when compared with pigs fed the MOD diet. Further analysis revealed no differences ($p > 0.05$) along the same predetermined white matter tracts in which pigs provided MOD diet exhibited higher FA, AD, or MD values when compared with pigs provided LOW diet.

3.2.3. Voxel-Based Morphometry

Voxel-based morphometry analysis identified differences in the location and size of tissue clusters between LOW and MOD dietary SL groups. Grey matter analysis revealed the largest and most significant cluster differences in which LOW pigs exhibited greater ($p < 0.05$) concentrations of grey matter when compared with MOD SL pigs (Table 1, Figure 4 and Figure S2 for full image set). These observed differences in which LOW > MOD were primarily localized to cortical tissue. Additionally, significant clusters revealed differences in cortical grey matter where MOD pigs exhibited larger concentrations when compared with LOW pigs; however, these clusters generally contained fewer voxels than the opposite comparison (i.e., MOD > LOW).

Table 1. Voxel-based morphometry comparison between pigs provided LOW and MOD dietary sialyllactose [1].

Tissue	Comparison	Anatomic Region [2]	Cluster (# Voxels)	Peak Level p-Value	Peak Level Pseudo-t	Local Maxima Coordinates [3] x	y	z
Grey	LOW > MOD	Lateral Ventricle/Corpus Callosum	141	<0.001	5.03	−4.9	14.0	7.0
		Right Cortex	1160	<0.001	4.5	9.1	10.5	−5.6
		Midbrain		0.001	4.02	−3.5	4.2	−9.8
		Midbrain/Right Cortex		0.007	2.8	7.7	2.8	−9.8
		Right Cortex	28	0.004	3.15	7.0	26.6	−2.8
		Left Cortex	163	0.004	3.13	−18.2	4.2	−2.1
	MOD > LOW	Left Cortex	139	<0.001	5.01	−14.7	4.2	11.9
		Right Cortex	39	0.001	3.74	12.6	0.7	11.9
		Left Cortex	23	0.004	3.1	−6.3	3.5	18.9
White	LOW > MOD	Caudate	128	0.001	3.95	2.1	18.9	2.8
		Midbrain/Right Cortex	93	0.001	3.74	7.7	3.5	−9.1
	MOD > LOW	Pons	147	<0.001	4.33	−6.3	−9.8	−9.1
		Left Cortex	32	0.007	2.85	−16.1	4.9	11.9
		Left Cortex	30	0.007	2.8	−12.6	0.7	12.6

[1] Voxel-based morphometry analysis of grey and white matter differences in the LOW ($n = 9$) and MOD ($n = 7$) pig brains. A threshold of $p < 0.01$ and minimum cluster size of 20 voxels was used to determine uncorrected p-values listed in the table. [2] Brain regions based on estimates from the University of Illinois Pig Brain Atlas [14]. [3] Local Maxima Coordinates: X increases from left (−) to right (+), y increases from posterior (−) to anterior (+) and z increases from inferior (−) to superior (+). Abbreviations: # (number of voxels).

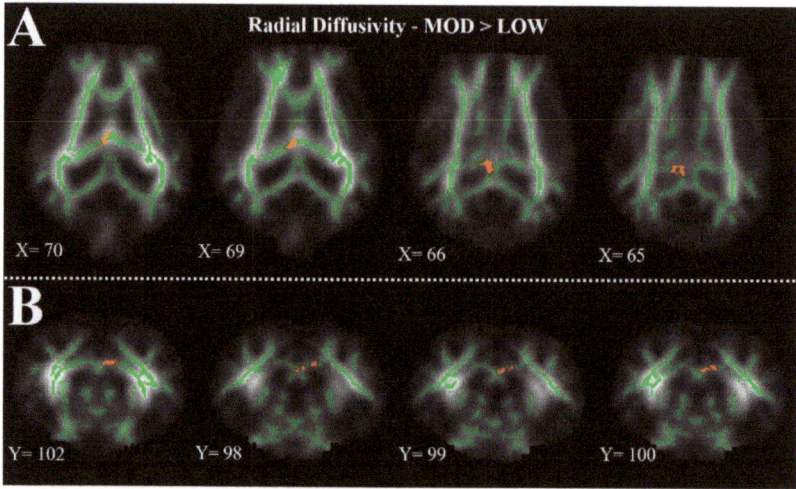

Figure 3. Tract-based spatial statistics (TBSS) illustrating differences in radial diffusivity (RD) between LOW and MOD dietary sialyllactose (SL) pigs. Pigs provided the MOD dietary SL treatment exhibited higher ($p < 0.05$) rates of radial diffusivity in the left hemisphere corpus callosum, when compared with LOW dietary SL pigs. The images generated from TBSS are and average of all LOW and MOD dietary SL pigs, green lines indicate regions in which all pigs exhibited white matter voxels. Representative slices were chosen to highlight areas in which RD values in MOD dietary SL pigs were significantly ($p < 0.05$) different compared with LOW dietary SL pigs. (**A**) Axial slices, with varying X-coordinates and static $Y = 120$ and $Z = 76$ coordinates, determined using University of Illinois Pig Brain Atlas [14]; (**B**) Coronal slices, with varying Y-coordinates and static $X = 73$ and $Z = 87$ coordinates, determined using the University of Illinois Pig Brain Atlas. Dark red and light red colors indicate degree of statistical differences from $p = 0.05$ to $p < 0.01$, respectively. For a more comprehensive image set of TBSS images the reader is referred to Supplemental Figure S1.

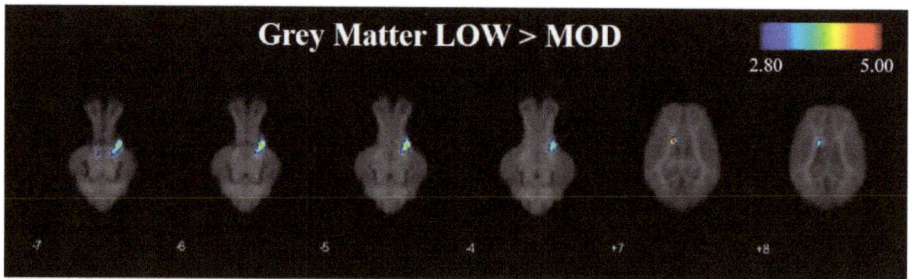

Figure 4. Voxel-based morphometry (VBM) heat maps illustrating grey matter tissue concentration differences between LOW and MOD dietary sialyllactose (SL) pigs. The colored bar indicates pseudo-t statistics, used to determine the *p*-uncorrected statistics provided in Table 1. Shown above are areas in which LOW dietary SL pigs exhibited greater ($p < 0.01$) concentrations of grey matter when compared with MOD dietary SL pigs. For a more comprehensive set of VBM images the reader is referred to Supplemental Figure S2.

Differences between LOW and MOD pig white matter concentrations were also evident, although these clusters contained fewer voxels than those observed in grey matter comparisons. Pigs provided the LOW diet exhibited higher ($p < 0.05$) concentrations of white matter in subcortical brain regions (i.e., caudate and midbrain) when compared with MOD pigs. Analysis of the reverse comparison (i.e., MOD > LOW) revealed that MOD pigs showed greater ($p < 0.05$) white matter concentrations in the pons and left cortex, compared with LOW pigs.

3.2.4. Brain Volumes

Due to excessive motion artifact in some of the acquired scans, the following number of pigs were analyzed per dietary treatment: CON ($n = 10$), LOW ($n = 9$), MOD ($n = 9$), HIGH ($n = 8$). No differences between absolute total brain volumes were observed between dietary treatments. Analysis of absolute volume in 19 different ROI did not result in differences due to diet (Table S1). Relative brain volume measures were generated by dividing an individual region of interest by the total brain volume, within subject and data is presented as a percent of total brain volume. No dietary effects were noted for relative brain volumes (Table S2). A trend ($p = 0.06$) for relative size of the left cortex was observed.

3.2.5. Single-Voxel Spectroscopy

Due to excessive motion artifact in some of the acquired scans the following number of pigs were analyzed per dietary treatment: CON ($n = 10$), LOW ($n = 9$), MOD ($n = 7$), HIGH ($n = 7$). Single-voxel spectroscopy revealed no difference due to diet in any of the seven measured metabolites. A trend for main effect of diet ($p = 0.07$) was observed for glutamate, with MOD pigs exhibiting numerically lower but not statistically significant, concentrations of glutamate when compared with all other groups (Table S3).

4. Discussion

Human milk OS are the third most abundant component in human milk and appear to be pivotal for proper neonatal development [4]. Approximately 10–30% of human milk OS are SA-containing, acidic OS, predominantly 3′-SL and 6′-SL [5,6]. Based on the high concentration of SL in human milk and the known roles of SA in brain development, there is interest in determining how dietary SL might influence neurodevelopment. This study assesses the effects of dietary SL on pig brain development using MRI and supports previous work assessing the effects of dietary SL on brain development in the biomedical pig model [17]. Results from this study indicate physiologically relevant levels of dietary SL influence SA tissue concentrations in the prefrontal cortex and hippocampus of young pigs, DTI measures in the corpus callosum and cortical grey and white matter tissue concentrations.

Supplementation of dietary compounds that contain SA have previously been reported to influence brain development but the ingredient used to supply SA varies widely. For example, dietary supplementation of casein glycomacropeptide, a SA-containing compound that is not a pure OS, increased learning and memory, raised cortical protein-bound SA concentrations and influenced the expression of learning-related genes in the five-week-old pig [18]. Moreover, intravenous infusion of C^{14}-labeled SA confirmed the ability of SA to cross the blood-brain-barrier and showed preferential accretion of labeled SA in the cortex of three-day-old pigs [19]. Provision of dietary SL has been shown to influence total SA and ganglioside-bound SA concentrations in the corpus callosum and cerebellum of three-week-old pigs [17]. Moreover, rats that were provided SA in the form of SL or galactosylated SA exhibited improved learning and increased brain SA and ganglioside concentrations compared with control rats [20]. A recent study suggested decreased stressor-induced anxiety-like behaviors in mice provided dietary SL compared with control mice [21]. These findings indicate an overt influence of dietary SA-containing compounds on the developing brain, however the optimal levels of supplementation and specific physiological effects of each compound remain to be elucidated.

Our study supplemented a modified whey protein enriched with a mixture of 3′-SL and 6′-SL at concentrations similar to mature sow milk (CON), mature bovine milk (LOW), 61-120 day human milk (MOD) and double what is typically found in mature human milk (HIGH) [4]. Notably, the LOW, MOD and HIGH dietary SL concentrations were formulated to be above the published concentrations of SL in infant formulas [4]. Analytical assessment conducted of the final diets indicated levels of

SL as follows: CON (55 mg SL/L), LOW (159 mg SL/L), MOD (429 mg/L) and HIGH (779 mg/L). These concentrations are likely due to inherent SL from bovine milk-derived ingredient sources used in the CON diet. The supplementation levels in the present study are lower compared with a recent pig study, which fed formula supplemented with pure forms of 3'-SL or 6'-SL at either 2 g/L or 4 g/L [17], which are greater than the SL concentrations of human colostrum [4]. To our knowledge, the study by Jacobi and colleagues and the present study are the only studies to assess the influence of dietary SL on brain development using the biomedical pig model.

4.1. Sialic Acid Concentrations

Analysis of SA in the prefrontal cortex indicated a greater proportion of bound SA in CON pigs when compared with LOW and MOD dietary SL pigs. Interestingly, concentrations of bound SA were not different between CON and HIGH dietary SL pigs. This study did not differentiate between SA bound to gangliosides or glycoproteins and it is unclear if the reduced concentration of bound SA in the LOW and MOD dietary SL groups is of physiological relevance. Results from Wang and colleagues [18] indicated slight increases in frontal cortex protein-bound SA when cGMP concentrations were 300, 635 and 830 mg/L compared with a 140 mg/L control and no differences in ganglioside-bound SA were noted between any treatment groups. When comparing our results (SL supplementation) with those from the study by Wang and colleagues (cGMP supplementation), it appears that structural specificity of dietary compounds that carry SA may be influential in SA accretion in the brain.

Herein, the ratio of free-to-bound SA indicated a higher proportion in the hippocampus of MOD pigs compared with CON and HIGH pigs but no difference between MOD and LOW pigs. Brain development is a heterogeneous process with brain regions developing at different rates [22]. It is known that the hippocampus is rapidly developing at 4-weeks of age in the pig [23] and research in chimpanzees indicates SA concentrations increase in the brain throughout development [11]. A study that supplemented three-day-old pigs with isotopically-labeled SA showed differences in brain region SA accretion after labeled SA injection, further suggesting region-specific accretion of SA during a highly dynamic period of neurodevelopment [19]. Wang and colleagues further suggest that the rate of SA accretion may be dependent on the species, subject age, dietary form of SA, and route of administration. Therefore, based on evidence from our study, we speculate that this increase in free SA relative to bound SA in the hippocampus could indicate a highly metabolic brain region that may be preparing SA to be incorporated into other compounds (e.g., glycoproteins or glycolipids) by preferentially partitioning free SA at the time of analysis. It is known that ganglioside concentrations in the brain rapidly increase perinatally [24], thus, future work should seek to characterize changes in free SA relative to bound SA in various brain regions over time to better understand the importance of this observation.

Assessment of total and free SA indicated no differences in their concentrations in the prefrontal cortex, cerebellum, or hippocampus. The lack of difference in total SA and free SA in these regions is in agreement with observations in a previous pig study, where researchers also did not observe differences in these regions in pigs that were provided pure forms of dietary SL [17]. While interesting, caution should be exercised when making comparisons between these two studies as the concentrations of dietary SL differed markedly, as described above. Notably, the lack of difference in blood SA concentrations may be explained through several different mechanisms. First, it is possible that circulating SA concentrations are tightly regulated in the body and endogenous synthesis of SA could have compensated for the difference in dietary SA. Additionally, it is possible that there is a limit at which dietary SA is bioavailable and the limit may have been met in each dietary treatment. Blood was only collected at the end of the study and it is also possible that differences in circulating SA concentrations existed earlier in the study but were corrected through compensatory mechanisms by the end of the study. Lastly, SL may have acted on gut microbiota and the microbiota may have influenced other circulating compounds which affected brain development. Future work should seek to quantify circulating SA concentrations at multiple time points, characterize bioavailability of dietary SA and assess the influence of the microbiome-gut-brain-axis.

4.2. Magnetic Resonance Imaging

Diffusion tensor imaging permits characterization of tissue microstructure through assessment of microscopic water movement in the brain [25]. Results from our study indicate differences due to dietary treatment in MD, AD and RD within the corpus callosum. Interestingly, for each measure, pigs that were provided MOD dietary SL exhibited the highest rates of diffusion across all diffusion measures. Moreover, for each diffusion measure (i.e., MD, AD and RD), pigs provided the HIGH dietary SL treatment exhibited reduced diffusivity when compared with the MOD dietary SL pigs. Provided the MOD dietary SL treatment was formulated to mimic mature human milk concentrations, it is possible that the HIGH dietary SL level (i.e., twice what is commonly observed in human milk) may not confer any added benefit to development. Although our pig study was not designed to look at specific morphology of brain structures, it is possible that the differences in diffusion properties between MOD and all other dietary treatments are a result of differences in corpus callosum structural architecture. A study of diffusion measures in the adult human corpus callosum indicates differences in fractional anisotropy among various sections of the corpus callosum [26]. These differences in diffusion values in the corpus callosum segments correspond to known structural differences (i.e., axon diameter, axon myelination and fiber packing) in each segment. Thus, future work should seek to characterize axon diameter, myelin thickness and density of fiber packing in the corpus callosum after a dietary SL intervention. While only trending, MD and RD in the left hippocampus indicated numerically higher rates of diffusion in the MOD dietary SL pigs compared with the CON, LOW and HIGH pigs. Interestingly, these observed trends for hippocampal MD and RD follow the same pattern as what was observed for free SA relative to bound SA concentrations in the hippocampus but it is unclear if the two are related. Also of note, the diffusion values observed across treatment groups in this study appear to be within the range of what has previously been reported and thus do not indicate any safety concerns.

The apparent sensitivity of the corpus callosum to dietary SL again support findings from a recent pig study, which showed increased ganglioside SA accretion in the corpus callosum of pigs supplemented with either 2 g/L 3′-SL or 6′-SL, compared with pigs receiving 4 g/L of 3′-SL or 6′-SL [17]. Despite the stark differences in dietary SL concentrations between the two studies, it is interesting to note that neither study observed linear increases in outcomes measures with higher supplementation rates. Jacobi and colleagues observed a quadratic effect for SL supplementation with the middle supplementation rate (i.e., 2 g SL/L compared with 0 g SL/L and 4 g SL/L) conferring the greatest total SA and ganglioside-bound SA accretion in the corpus callosum. Although we did not statistically test quadratic effects, anecdotally, similar patterns were observed with the MOD dietary SL group exhibiting the highest rates of diffusion relative to CON, LOW and HIGH dietary SL pigs. Together these findings may suggest an optimal window at which dietary SL modulates corpus callosum development.

To better characterize the observations of corpus callosum DTI findings, we also assessed the difference between the LOW and MOD dietary SL treatments using TBSS. Tract-based spatial statistics provides a visual comparison between treatment groups, thereby elucidating areas within white matter tracts where structural differences may exist. From the heat maps generated in this analysis, it is clear that the largest differences in RD of the corpus callosum exist in the left hemisphere. A study of two-year-old chimpanzee cortical brain tissue indicates greater SA accretion in the left hemisphere compared with the right hemisphere [11]. Although this study did not assess corpus callosum SA enrichment, these findings, coupled with the diffusion trends in the left hippocampus and left hemisphere corpus callosum TBSS observations, might suggest sensitivity of the left hemisphere to dietary forms of SA early in life. Also of note, the SA tissue quantification was performed on right hemisphere samples. Provided the results presented above and work by Wang and colleagues [11], it is possible that more robust dietary effects may have been observed in left hemisphere tissue analyses.

To further investigate differences in grey and white matter development, VBM was used to compare tissue concentrations between LOW and MOD dietary SL pigs. Pigs that were provided the LOW dietary SL treatment appeared to have greater concentrations of grey matter in the right cortex and the midbrain when compared with MOD dietary SL pigs. Conversely, assessment of pigs provided the MOD diet appeared to have areas of increased grey matter in localized areas of left cortex when compared with LOW dietary SL pigs. It is known that grey matter tissue concentrations change throughout development [27], however it is unclear if these changes may be due to axonal growth or synaptic pruning, each of which may influence grey matter tissue concentrations. Future work should seek to characterize markers of synaptic pruning and axon growth to better understand if decreased tissue concentrations in MOD dietary SL pigs may be a result of pruning or growth events.

4.3. Limitations

A recent study of porcine milk OS suggests 3′-SL is the predominant acidic OS with a concentration of 100 mg/L in colostrum that falls below 50 mg/L by day 7 of lactation [8]. Provided the low concentrations of 3′-SL and undetectable concentrations of 6′-SL in porcine milk, it is possible that all concentrations of dietary SL used in this study were sufficient to support normal brain development and future work should seek to compare with a control diet which does not contain endogenous SL. Additionally, it remains unclear exactly how SL is digested and absorbed into the body. The findings presented herein may be a result of dietary SL directly providing SA for brain development. However, recent evidence in the pig model suggests alterations in gut development may modulate particular aspects of brain development [28], therefore it is also possible that dietary SL may have stimulated gut development which in turn influenced brain development. In fact, dietary SL has been shown to alter proximal and distal colon microbiota in the pig [17], thus it is possible dietary SL may influence the brain through the gut-brain-axis. Future work should seek to characterize the metabolism of dietary SL and elucidate its main mode of influence in brain development. Also of note, a rat model of necrotizing enterocolitis showed a structure-dependent response to a specific SA-containing OS, thereby suggesting unique roles for each isomer of SA-containing OS [29]. This finding in the gut coupled with varying effects of SA-containing molecules in the brain suggest structure specific functions of SA molecules and their role in infant development. Therefore, future work should seek to sensitively characterize the unique role of individual dietary SA containing compounds, in order to elucidate their specific physiological relevance.

5. Conclusions

There is a lack of studies directly assessing the influence of dietary SL on brain development. The data from our study adds to a growing body of literature, which suggests brain development is sensitive to the presence of SL in the diet. To our knowledge, this is the first study to use magnetic resonance imaging to quantify differences in brain development due to dietary SL. Moreover, this study substantiates recent findings that the corpus callosum and left hemisphere appear to be influenced by the presence of SL in the diet.

Supplementary Materials: The following are available online at www.mdpi.com/2072-6643/9/12/1297/s1, Table S1: Dietary sialyllactose does not influence absolute brain volumes; Table S2: Dietary sialyllactose does not influence relative brain volumes; Table S3: Dietary sialyllactose does not affect single-voxel spectroscopy measures; Figure S1: LOW and MOD pigs exhibit differences in tract-based spatial statistics; Figure S2: LOW and MOD pigs exhibit differences in grey and white matter concentrations.

Acknowledgments: The authors would like to thank Mead Johnson Pediatric Nutrition for providing the grant funding and the diet to perform this study. The authors would like to thank Nancy Dodge, Holly Tracy and Tracy Henigman from the Beckman Imaging Center for their help with neuroimaging procedures. The authors would also like to thank Kristen Karkiewicz for pig rearing and day-to-day pig operations. The authors acknowledge the efforts of Mead Johnson Nutrition employees, Shireen Doultani and Julieta Ortiz for their assistance with formulating and manufacturing the pig diets. Lastly, the authors would like to thank Misha Ahmad for her help in pig neuroimaging data preparation.

Author Contributions: M.C., B.M.B., S.M.D. and R.N.D. were involved in conceptualizing and planning the study. A.T.M., S.A.F., S.M.D. and R.N.D. were involved in study implementation. A.T.M., S.A.F., B.L., S.M.D. and R.N.D. were involved in data analysis and interpretation. All authors were involved in manuscript preparation and have read and approved of the final manuscript.

Conflicts of Interest: S.M.D. and R.N.D. were received grant funding from Mead Johnson Nutrition. B.L., M.C., B.M.B. were employees of Mead Johnson Nutrition throughout the duration of this study.

References

1. Ballard, O.; Morrow, A.L. Human milk composition: Nutrients and bioctive factors. *Pediatr. Clin. N. Am.* **2013**, *60*, 1–24. [CrossRef] [PubMed]

2. Martin, C.R.; Ling, P.-R.; Blackburn, G.L. Review of infant feeding: Key features of breast milk and infant formula. *Nutrients* **2016**, *8*, 279. [CrossRef] [PubMed]

3. Bode, L. Human milk oligosaccharides: Every baby needs a sugar mama. *Glycobiology* **2017**, *22*, 1147–1162. [CrossRef] [PubMed]

4. Ten Bruggencate, S.J.; Bovee-Oudenhoven, I.M.; Feitsma, A.L.; van Hoffen, E.; Schoterman, M.H. Functional role and mechanisms of sialyllactose and other sialylated milk oligosaccharides. *Nutr. Rev.* **2014**, *72*, 377–389. [CrossRef] [PubMed]

5. Ninonuevo, M.R.; Park, Y.; Yin, H.; Zhang, J.; Ward, R.E.; Clowers, B.H.; German, J.B.; Freeman, S.L.; Killeen, K.; Grimm, R.; et al. A strategy for annotating the human milk glycome. *J. Agric. Food Chem.* **2006**, *54*, 7471–7480. [CrossRef] [PubMed]

6. Martin-Sosa, S.; Martin, M.; Garcia-Prado, L.; Hueso, P. Sialyloligosaccharides in human and bovine milk and in infant formulas: Variations with the progression of lactation. *J. Dairy Sci.* **2003**, *86*, 52–59. [CrossRef]

7. Urashima, T.; Saito, T.; Nakamura, T.; Messer, M. Oligosaccharides of milk and colostrum in non-human mammals. *Glycoconj. J.* **2001**, *18*, 357–371. [CrossRef] [PubMed]

8. Mudd, A.T.; Salcedo, J.; Alexander, L.S.; Johnson, S.K.; Getty, C.M.; Chichlowski, M.; Berg, B.M.; Barile, D.; Dilger, R.N. Porcine milk oligosaccharides and sialic acid concentrations vary throughout lactation. *Front. Nutr.* **2016**, *3*, 39. [CrossRef] [PubMed]

9. Schnaar, R.L.; Gerardy-Schahn, R.; Hildebrandt, H. Sialic acids in the brain: Gangliosides and polysialic acid in nervous system development, stability, disease, and regeneration. *Physiol. Rev.* **2014**, *94*, 461–518. [CrossRef] [PubMed]

10. Wang, B.; McVeagh, P.; Petocz, P.; Brand-Miller, J. Brain ganglioside and glycoprotein sialic acid in breastfed compared with formula-fed infants. *Am. J. Clin. Nutr.* **2003**, *78*, 1024–1029. [PubMed]

11. Wang, B.; Miller, J.B.; McNeil, Y.; McVeagh, P. Sialic acid concentration of brain gangliosides: Variation among eight mammalian species. *Comp. Biochem. Physiol.* **1998**, *119*, 435–439. [CrossRef]

12. Mudd, A.T.; Dilger, R.N. Early-Life nutrition and neurodevelopment: Use of the piglet as a translational model. *Adv. Nutr.* **2017**, *8*, 92–104. [CrossRef] [PubMed]

13. Mudd, A.T.; Getty, C.; Sutton, B.; Dilger, R. Perinatal choline deficiency delays brain development and alters metabolite concentrations in the young pig. *Nutr. Neurosci.* **2016**, *19*, 425–433. [CrossRef] [PubMed]

14. Conrad, M.S.; Sutton, B.P.; Dilger, R.N.; Johnson, R. An in vivo three-dimensional magnetic resonance imaging-based averaged brain collection of the neonatal piglet (*Sus scrofa*). *PLoS ONE* **2014**, *9*, e107650. [CrossRef] [PubMed]

15. Radlowski, E.C.; Conrad, M.S.; Lezmi, S.; Dilger, R.N.; Sutton, B.; Larsen, R.; Johnson, R.W. A neonatal piglet model for investigating brain and cognitive development in small for gestational age human infants. *PLoS ONE* **2014**, *9*, e91951. [CrossRef] [PubMed]

16. Mudd, A.; Alexander, L.; Berding, K.; Waworuntu, R.; Berg, B.; Donovan, S.; Dilger, R. Dietary prebiotics, milk fat globule membrane and lactoferrin affects structural neurodevelopment in the young piglet. *Front. Pediatr.* **2016**, *4*, 1–10. [CrossRef] [PubMed]

17. Jacobi, S.K.; Yatsunenko, T.; Li, D.; Dasgupta, S.; Yu, R.K.; Berg, B.M.; Chichlowski, M.; Odle, J. Dietary isomers of sialyllactose increase ganglioside sialic acid concentrations in the corpus callosum and cerebellum and modulate the colonic microbiota of formula-fed piglets. *J. Nutr.* **2016**, *146*, 200–208. [CrossRef] [PubMed]

18. Wang, B.; Yu, B.; Karim, M.; Hu, H.; Sun, Y.; McGreevy, P.; Petocz, P.; Held, S.; Brand-Miller, J. Dietary sialic acid supplementation improves learning and memory in piglets. *Am. J. Clin. Nutr.* **2007**, *85*, 561–569. [PubMed]

19. Wang, B.; Downing, J.A.; Petocz, P.; Brand-Miller, J.; Bryden, W.L. Metabolic fate of intravenously administered *N*-acetylneuraminic acid-6-14C in newborn piglets. *Asia Pac. J. Clin. Nutr.* **2007**, *16*, 110–115. [PubMed]

20. Sakai, F.; Ikeuchi, Y.; Urashima, T.; Fujihara, M.; Ohtsuki, K.; Yanahira, S. Effects of feeding sialyllactose and galactosylated *N*-acetylneuraminic acid on swimming learning ability and brain lipid composition in adult rats. *J. Appl. Glycosci.* **2006**, *53*, 249–254. [CrossRef]

21. Tarr, A.J.; Galley, J.D.; Fisher, S.E.; Chichlowski, M.; Berg, B.M.; Bailey, M.T. The prebiotics 3′Sialyllactose and 6′Sialyllactose diminish stressor-induced anxiety-like behavior and colonic microbiota alterations: Evidence for effects on the gut-brain axis. *Brain Behav. Immun.* **2015**, *50*, 166–177. [CrossRef] [PubMed]

22. Deoni, S.C.L.; Mercure, E.; Blasi, A.; Gasston, D.; Thomson, A.; Johnson, M.; Williams, S.C.R.; Murphy, D.G.M. Mapping infant brain myelination with magnetic resonance imaging. *J. Neurosci.* **2011**, *31*, 784–791. [CrossRef] [PubMed]

23. Conrad, M.S.; Dilger, R.N.; Johnson, R.W. Brain growth of the domestic pig (*Sus scrofa*) from 2 to 24 weeks of age: A longitudinal MRI study. *Dev. Neurosci.* **2012**, *34*, 291–298. [CrossRef] [PubMed]

24. Wang, B. Sialic acid is an essential nutrient for brain development and cognition. *Annu. Rev. Nutr.* **2009**, *29*, 177–222. [CrossRef] [PubMed]

25. Alexander, A.L.; Lee, J.E.; Lazar, M.; Field, A.S. Diffusion tensor imaging of the brain. *Neurotherapeutics* **2007**, *4*, 316–329. [CrossRef] [PubMed]

26. Hofer, S.; Frahm, J. Topography of the human corpus callosum revisited-Comprehensive fiber tractography using diffusion tensor magnetic resonance imaging. *Neuroimage* **2006**, *32*, 989–994. [CrossRef] [PubMed]

27. Knickmeyer, R.C.; Gouttard, S.; Kang, C.; Evans, D.; Wilber, K.; Smith, J.K.; Hamer, R.M.; Lin, W.; Gerig, G.; Gilmore, J.H. A structural MRI study of human brain development from birth to 2 years. *J. Neurosci.* **2008**, *28*, 12176–12182. [CrossRef] [PubMed]

28. Mudd, A.T.; Berding, K.; Wang, M.; Donovan, S.M.; Dilger, R.N. Serum cortisol mediates the relationship between fecal Ruminococcus & brain *N*-acetylaspartate in the young pig. *Gut Microbes* **2017**, 1–12. [CrossRef]

29. Jantscher-krenn, E.; Zherebtsov, M.; Nissan, C.; Goth, K. The human milk oligosaccharide disialyllacto-*N*-tetraose prevents necrotising enterocolitis in neonatal rats. *Gut* **2014**, *61*, 1417–1425. [CrossRef] [PubMed]

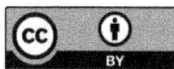

© 2017 by the authors. Licensee MDPI, Basel, Switzerland. This article is an open access article distributed under the terms and conditions of the Creative Commons Attribution (CC BY) license (http://creativecommons.org/licenses/by/4.0/).

nutrients

MDPI

Article

Early-Life Iron Deficiency Reduces Brain Iron Content and Alters Brain Tissue Composition Despite Iron Repletion: A Neuroimaging Assessment

Austin T. Mudd [1,2,*], Joanne E. Fil [1,2], Laura C. Knight [1,3], Fan Lam [4], Zhi-Pei Liang [4,5] and Ryan N. Dilger [1,2,3,4,6,*]

[1] Piglet Nutrition & Cognition Laboratory, University of Illinois Urbana-Champaign, Urbana, IL 61801, USA; jfil2@illinois.edu (J.E.F.); knight24@illinois.edu (L.C.K.)
[2] Neuroscience Program, University of Illinois Urbana-Champaign, Urbana, IL 61801, USA
[3] Division of Nutrition Sciences, University of Illinois Urbana-Champaign, Urbana, IL 61801, USA
[4] Beckman Institute for Advanced Science & Technology, University of Illinois Urbana-Champaign, Urbana, IL 61801, USA; fanlam1@illinois.edu (F.L.); z-liang@illinois.edu (Z.-P.L.)
[5] Department of Electrical & Computer Engineering, University of Illinois Urbana-Champaign, Urbana, IL 61801, USA
[6] Department of Animal Sciences, University of Illinois Urbana-Champaign, Urbana, IL 61801, USA
* Correspondence: amudd2@illinois.edu (A.T.M.); rdilger2@illinois.edu (R.N.D.)

Received: 20 December 2017; Accepted: 25 January 2018; Published: 27 January 2018

Abstract: Early-life iron deficiency has lifelong influences on brain structure and cognitive function, however characterization of these changes often requires invasive techniques. There is a need for non-invasive assessment of early-life iron deficiency with potential to translate findings to the human clinical setting. In this study, 28 male pigs were provided either a control diet (CONT; $n = 14$; 23.5 mg Fe/L milk replacer) or an iron-deficient diet (ID; $n = 14$; 1.56 mg Fe/L milk replacer) for phase 1 of the study, from postnatal day (PND) 2 until 32. Twenty pigs ($n = 10$/diet from phase 1 were used in phase 2 of the study from PND 33 to 61, where all pigs were provided a common iron-sufficient diet, regardless of their phase 1 dietary iron status. All pigs were subjected to magnetic resonance imaging at PND 32 and again at PND 61, and quantitative susceptibility mapping was used to assess brain iron content at both imaging time-points. Data collected on PND 61 were analyzed using voxel-based morphometry and tract-based spatial statistics to determine tissue concentration difference and white matter tract integrity, respectively. Quantitative susceptibility mapping outcomes indicated reduced iron content in the pons, medulla, cerebellum, left cortex, and left hippocampus of ID pigs compared with CONT pigs, regardless of imaging time-point. In contrast, iron contents were increased in the olfactory bulbs of ID pigs compared with CONT pigs. Voxel-based morphometric analysis indicated increased grey and white matter concentrations in CONT pigs compared with ID pigs that were evident at PND 61. Differences in tissue concentrations were predominately located in cortical tissue as well as the cerebellum, thalamus, caudate, internal capsule, and hippocampi. Tract-based spatial statistics indicated increased fractional anisotropy values along subcortical white matter tracts in CONT pigs compared with ID pigs that were evident on PND 61. All described differences were significant at $p \leq 0.05$. Results from this study indicate that neuroimaging can sensitively detect structural and physiological changes due to early-life iron deficiency, including grey and white matter volumes, iron contents, as well as reduced subcortical white matter integrity, despite a subsequent period of dietary iron repletion.

Keywords: neurodevelopment; iron deficiency; pig; iron repletion; myelination; pediatric nutrition; brain iron

1. Introduction

Iron deficiency is the most common micronutrient deficiency worldwide [1,2] and a deficiency during the perinatal period has lifelong implications. Infants are at an increased risk for iron deficiency [3] and the developing brain is highly vulnerable to alterations in iron status [4–7]. Research in humans has shown that iron deficiency early in life results in delayed motor development by ten months of age [8], delayed cognitive processing by ten years of age [9], altered recognition memory and executive functions at 19 years of age [10], and poorer emotional health in the mid-twenties [11]. It is clear that early-life iron deficiency has lasting effects on cognitive performance, yet it remains to be elucidated what structural differences in brain development might underlie these persistent cognitive changes. Some studies in humans have used other non-invasive techniques such as evoked potential recordings [12], electrophysiological recording and processing [9] and electroencephalography [13] to explain structural alterations in brain development related to iron deficiency. While these methods may potentially explain a mechanism for altered brain development, more sensitive assessments are needed to non-invasively characterize the brain regions influenced by iron deficiency.

The presence of iron in the brain is necessary for proper vascular development [14], myelination [15], neurotransmitter synthesis [16,17], and neuron morphology [18,19]. To date, many of the mechanisms for iron's involvement in brain development have been determined using invasive techniques in animal models. While necessary and informative, these methods are not feasible in clinical populations, thus there is a need to characterize similar findings using non-invasive techniques. Magnetic resonance imaging (MRI) is one method that may bridge the gap between invasive techniques used in animal models and cognitive and surface recording assessments used in humans. A recent study indicated maternal iron status and cord blood ferritin measures related to markers of infant brain development, which were assessed using diffusion tensor imaging [20]. While this finding is informative, hematological indices of iron status often do not predict brain iron content, as the brain tends to deplete prior to blood tissue [5]. Thus, a non-invasive assessment of brain iron is needed to quantify iron levels throughout development, thereby illuminating differences that may not be predicted by hematological indices. Quantitative susceptibility mapping (QSM) is an MRI method that has been used to quantify altered iron status in clinical cases of restless leg syndrome [21] and β-thalassemia [22]; thus, it is possible that these methods may be able to sensitively detect altered brain iron status in cases of dietary iron deficiency. In fact, a recent neuroimaging study that used QSM in children found that brain iron content in the caudate nucleus related to performance on spatial intelligence quotient tests [23], thereby offering insight into brain regions that may underlie cognitive differences due to iron status. Moreover, neuroimaging allows for assessment of structural brain development such as myelination, and grey matter and white matter tissue distributions, and may prove useful in sensitively characterizing structural differences later in life.

We previously reported that early-life iron deficiency resulted in decreased relative brain volumes of specific regions and region-specific reductions in diffusion tensor measures, which persisted in developing pig brains even after a subsequent period of dietary iron repletion [24]. Interestingly, these differences in microstructural brain development were present at postnatal day (PND) 61 despite a lack of difference in absolute brain volume between iron-deficient (ID) and control (CONT) pigs at that time-point. These findings suggest comprehensively assessing the effects of iron deficiency is necessary to elucidate region-specific, rather than whole brain, implications of altered nutrient status. To further expand upon our previous findings, herein we analyzed differences between early-life ID and control CONT pigs in concentrations of brain grey matter, white matter, and measures of white matter tract development at PND 61. Due to the highly dynamic nature of the developing brain and the influence of iron on myelin and neuron morphology, we hypothesized that grey and white matter tissue concentrations would be altered by early life iron status and remain evident at PND 61. Thus, the aim of this study was to identify specific regions of the brain that remained structurally different in ID pigs after a subsequent period of iron repletion Additionally we used, a non-invasive neuroimaging technique, QSM, to characterize changes in brain iron content. Using this method, we hypothesized that piglets provided an ID diet early in life would exhibit decreased iron content in the brain, as measured through QSM.

2. Materials and Methods

2.1. Animal Care and Housing

Twenty-eight, naturally-farrowed, intact male pigs were obtained from Carthage Veterinary Services and transferred to the University of Illinois Piglet Nutrition and Cognition Laboratory (PNCL) at PND 2. Per standard agricultural protocol, pigs were provided an intramuscular injection of a prophylactic antibiotic (0.1 mL of ceftiofur crystalline free acid (Exceed, Zoetis, Parsippany, NJ, USA)) within 24 h of birth. Contrary to typical agricultural procedures, pigs on this study were not administered an intramuscular injection of iron dextran because iron was the nutrient being manipulated as per the experimental design. Recent pig studies observed hippocampal transcriptome changes [25] and possible effects of iron overload [26] after a bolus administration of iron dextran in the first few days of life, which further justifies our decision to not provide iron dextran to any pigs. Upon arrival to PNCL on PND 2, pigs were stratified into one of two experimental diets, described below. Pigs were randomly allocated into treatment groups to account for initial bodyweight and maternal genetics, with no bodyweight or iron status differences between the groups at the start of the study. Pigs were provided experimental milk replacer diets from PND 2 until PND 32 (phase 1), at which point both treatment groups were weaned onto a series of nutritionally-adequate diets from PND 33 until PND 61 (phase 2). A detailed description of phase 1 and phase 2 rearing environments has been previously described [24]. All animal and experimental procedures were in accordance with the National Research Council Guide for the Care and Use of Laboratory Animals and approved by the University of Illinois at Urbana-Champaign Institutional Animal Care and Use Committee. Approval for this research project was confirmed on 3 March 2015 and is identified as IACUC 15034 at the University of Illinois Urbana-Champaign.

2.2. Dietary Treatments

For phase 1 of this study, pigs ($N = 28$; $n = 14$ per diet) were provided one of two dietary treatments with varying iron content. The CONT diet was formulated to meet all of the nutrient requirements of the growing pig and was formulated to contain 117.5 mg Fe/kg milk replacer powder. The ID diet was similar to the CONT diet, however iron was only formulated to be supplemented at 7.8 mg Fe/kg milk replacer powder. Additionally, both diets were formulated to contain arachidonic acid (ARA) (2.08 g ARA/kg milk replacer powder) and docosahexanoeic acid (DHA) (1.04 g DHA/kg milk replacer powder). Milk replacer was reconstituted fresh daily with 200 g of milk replacer powder per 800 g water. Thus, formulated iron concentrations in reconstituted pig milk replacers were: CONT, 23.5 mg Fe/L milk replacer, and ID, 1.56 mg Fe/L milk replacer. All pigs were provided ad libitum access to liquid diets from PND 2 until PND 32.

For phase 2 of this study, all pigs ($N = 20$, $n = 10$/phase 1 diet) were weaned onto the same series of age-appropriate, nutritionally-adequate solid diets, regardless of their phase 1 dietary iron status. Pigs were provided ad libitum access to water and standard complex diets (major ingredients including corn, whey, and soybean meal) and standard agricultural feeding practices were followed by sequentially switching from stage 1 diets, to stage 2 diets, to stage 3 diets, on PND 33, 41, and 50 respectively. During this phase of the study, all diets were formulated to meet all nutrient requirements of the growing pig [27], including iron. No zinc oxide, copper sulfate, or in-feed antibiotics were included in any diets.

2.3. Magnetic Resonance Imaging

All pigs remaining in each phase underwent MRI procedures on PND 32 or 33 for phase 1 and again at PND 61 or 62 for phase 2, at the Beckman Institute for Advanced Science and Technology

Biomedical Imaging Center. For phase 1, 28 pigs (n = 14 per diet) were subjected to neuroimaging procedures and for phase 2, 20 pigs (n = 10 per phase 1 diet) were subjected to neuroimaging procedures. Imaging procedures were performed using a Siemens MAGNETOM Trio 3T scanner (Siemens, Erlangen, Germany), with a custom pig-specific 8-channel head coil at PND 32 and a human 8-channel head coil at PND 61. Upon arrival to the imaging facility, anesthesia was induced using an intramuscular injection of telazol: ketamine: xylazine solution [50.0 mg tiletamine plus 50.0 mg of zolazepam reconstituted with 2.50 mL ketamine (100 g/L) and 2.50 mL xylazine (100 g/L); Fort Dodge Animal Health] administered at 0.03 mL/kg body weight, and maintained with inhalation of isoflurane (98% O_2, 2% isoflurane). Pigs were immobilized during all MRI procedures. Visual observation of each pig's well-being, as well as observations of heart rate, PO_2 and percent of isoflurane were recorded every 5 min. during the procedure. Total scan time for each pig was approximately 60 min. Upon completion of the scan, pig respiration and heart rate were monitored every 15 min. until complete recovery from anesthesia. Imaging techniques are briefly described below.

2.3.1. Structural MRI Acquisition & Analysis

A T_1-weighted magnetization-prepared rapid gradient echo (MPRAGE) sequence was used to obtain anatomic images of the pig brain, with a 0.7 mm isotropic voxel size. The following specific parameters were used for the MPRAGE sequence: repetition time (TR) = 1900 ms; echo time (TE) = 2.49 ms; inversion time (TI) = 900 ms; 224 slices; field of view (FOV) = 180 × 180 mm^2; flip angle = 9°. Pig brains were manually extracted as previously described [28]. All toolboxes described herein were available in SPM12 (Wellcome Department of Clinical Neurology, London, UK) and Matlab R2015a was used for data processing. Once extracted, the 'Coregister: Estimate & Reslice' toolbox was used to coregister individual brains to the Pig MRI Atlas [29]. Next, the 'Old Normalize: Estimate & Reslice' toolbox was used to transform individual pig brains into atlas space. The following parameters in Old Normalize were used for pig specific data processing: template image (Pig MRI Atlas), bounding box (−30.1 −35 −28/30.1 44.8 31.5), voxel size (0.7). The "Segment" function of SPM12 and pig-specific prior probability tissue maps were then used to segment the brains into grey matter and white matter. Voxel-based morphometry (VBM) analysis was performed to assess grey and white matter tissue concentrations using SPM12 software. The Diffeomorphic Anatomical Registration using Exponentiated Lie Algebra (DARTEL) toolbox was used with pig-specific specifications that included changing the bounding box of −30.1 to 30.1, −35 to 44.8, −28 to 31.5; and a voxel size of 0.7 mm^3. After the nonlinear transformation of the data in the DARTEL procedure, flow fields were created and converted to warp files. The warp files generated were then applied to the subject's grey and white matter. The modulated data were smoothed with a 4 mm full-width half maximum, and were subjected to VBM procedures using the SPM12 toolbox.

2.3.2. Quantitative Susceptibility Mapping

Brain tissue susceptibility was obtained to access the iron content change due to iron-deficiency. To this end, whole brain ^1H magnetic resonance spectroscopic imaging (MRSI) data without water suppression were acquired using the recently proposed spectroscopic imaging by exploiting spatiospectral correlation SPICE-based acquisition [30,31]. Without water suppression, QSM of brain tissues can be extracted from the phase information encoded in the water spectroscopic signals [31,32]. The detailed acquisition parameters are as follows: TR/TE = 310/4 ms, FOV = 200 × 160 × 64 mm^3, matrix size = 100 × 120 × 26, flip angle = 37°, readout bandwidth = 167 kHz, number of echoes acquired each TR = 200, and echo spacing = 850 ms. Susceptibility maps were extracted from the water spectroscopic data using the following algorithm (see Peng et al., 2017 [31] for more details): (1) total B_0 field inhomogeneity maps were estimated by using a voxel-by-voxel least-squares fitting of the multi-echo data; (2) the tissue susceptibility induced field inhomogeneity was extracted from the total field by solving the Laplacian boundary value problem [33]; (3) susceptibility maps were then determined by solving the tissue field to susceptibility dipole inversion [32]; and (4) regional susceptibility values were obtained by averaging the susceptibility values in different regions of interest ROIs, using the University of Illinois Piglet Brain Atlas [29] (http://pigmri.illinois.edu/).

2.3.3. Tract-Based Spatial Statistics

Diffusion tensor imaging was used to assess white matter maturation and axonal tract integrity using a b-value = 1000 s/mm^2 across 30 directions and a 2 mm isotropic voxel. Diffusion-weighted echoplanar imaging EPI images were assessed in FMRIB Software Library (FSL) for fractional anisotropy (FA), mean diffusivity (MD), axial diffusivity (AD), and radial diffusivity (RD) using methods previously described [28]. The FSL 5.0 toolbox was used for tract-based spatial statistics (TBSS) assessment of FA data [34,35]. Fractional anisotropy images, previously generated from diffusion data, were manually extracted, and all FA data from individual subjects were aligned using the FSL nonlinear registration tool FNIRT. Upon alignment, the study-specific mean FA image was created and a mean FA skeleton representing the center of all common tracts was established. A threshold of 0.2 was determined to be sensitive for mean FA tract delineation. Once the study-specific mean FA skeleton was created, each subjects' aligned FA data were projected onto the mean FA skeleton and the resulting voxel-wise cross-subject data were used for statistical analyses [34,35]. For all TBSS analyses involving registration to an atlas, the University of Illinois Piglet Brain Atlas (http://pigmri.illinois.edu/) was used in place of human brain templates [29].

2.4. Statistical Analysis

All researchers involved in this study (i.e., those performing daily procedures, data collection, and data analysis steps) remained blinded to dietary treatment identity until final data analyses had been completed. Data were analyzed by using the MIXED procedure of SAS 9.4 (SAS Institute, Cary, NC, USA). Quantitative susceptibility measures were analyzed from data generated at PND 32 and 61, thus all data were analyzed using a 2-way repeated measures analysis of variance (ANOVA) (i.e., dietary iron status with postnatal day at time of neuroimaging acquisition as the repeated measure). Interactive effects were defined as an interaction between diet (CONT vs. ID) and MRI day (PND 32 vs. 61). The number of animals per treatment group was based on a power analysis using the variability estimates from previous studies to detect differences with sufficient power of 80% and at a significance of 0.05. Data were analyzed for outliers (defined as having a studentized residual with an absolute value greater than 3) and outliers were removed prior to statistical analysis. Significance was accepted at $p \leq 0.05$. Data are presented as least-squares means with pooled standard errors of the mean (SEM).

2.4.1. Voxel-Based Morphometry Statistics

Voxel-based morphometry analyses were performed on data acquired at PND 61. As such, two-sample permutation t-tests were performed on a voxel-by-voxel basis for grey and white matter volume differences between animals on the early-life CONT and ID diets, with an uncorrected $p < 0.001$. An additional threshold criterion of at least 20 edge-connected voxels was used.

2.4.2. Tract-Based Spatial Statistics

For TBSS analysis, only data acquired at PND 61 was analyzed. A nonparametric permutation inference function called 'randomise' was used within the FSL toolbox and run as a two-sample t-test with 500 permutations to compare the effects of early-life CONT and ID diets. Multiple comparisons were also accounted for within the randomize function. The resulting statistical analysis was then presented as heat maps indicating brain areas where FA values differed between dietary treatments.

3. Results

3.1. Quantitative Susceptibility Mapping

Interactive effects of diet and MRI day were not observed for region-specific QSM measures. A main effect of dietary treatment (i.e., independent of MRI day) ($p < 0.05$) was observed in the pons, medulla, cerebellum, left cortex, olfactory bulb, and left hippocampus, Figure 1 and Table 1. Regardless of imaging time-point, pigs receiving the ID diet exhibited lower QSM values in the pons ($p < 0.001$), medulla ($p = 0.02$), cerebellum ($p < 0.01$), left cortex ($p < 0.01$), and left hippocampus ($p < 0.001$) when compared with CONT pigs. Conversely, pigs on the ID diet exhibited higher ($p = 0.04$) QSM values in the olfactory bulb when compared with CONT pigs, regardless of imaging time-point.

A main effect of MRI day (i.e., independent of early-life iron status) ($p < 0.05$) was observed for corpus callosum, hypothalamus, and right cortex. The QSM measures in the corpus callosum ($p = 0.03$) increased from 0.26 ± 1.36 ppb on PND 32 to 4.89 ± 1.36 ppb at PND 61. In the right cortex, QSM measures increased ($p = 0.03$) from -1.83 ± 0.42 ppb on PND 32 to -0.21 ± 0.42 ppb at PND 61. Conversely, the QSM measures in hypothalamus decreased ($p = 0.04$) from -3.65 ± 1.70 ppb on PND 32 to -8.62 ± 1.70 ppb on PND 61. Notably, as iron content increases, QSM measures change from negative (i.e., indicating diamagnetic tissue properties) to positive (i.e., indicating paramagnetic tissue properties). Note, no interactive effects were observed, but means for both dietary treatments at both imaging time points are presented in Table 1. Accordingly, a main effect of diet can be determined by averaging the measures within dietary treatment group for each brain region and a main effect of time can be determined by averaging the two treatment groups at each imaging time point.

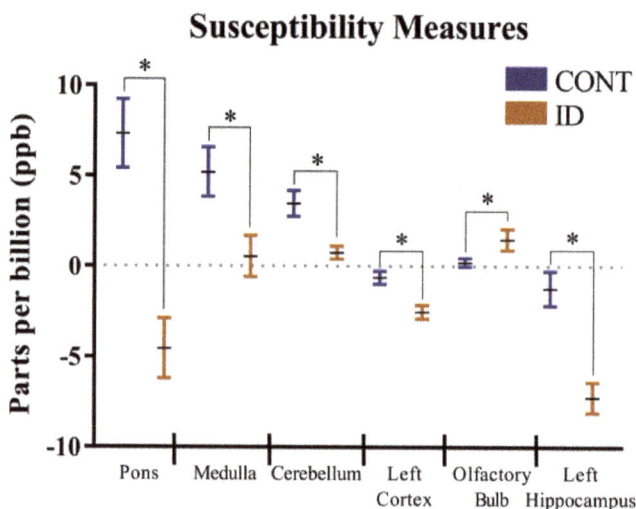

Figure 1. Measures of average iron content in brain regions were influenced by dietary iron status, regardless of imaging time-point. Because there was no significant interaction between diet and magnetic resonance imaging (MRI) day, this figure only shows the significant main effects of diet, regardless of time. Reduced iron content in the pons ($p < 0.001$), medulla ($p = 0.018$), cerebellum ($p = 0.005$), left cortex ($p = 0.004$), and left hippocampus ($p < 0.001$) was observed in ID pigs compared with CONT pigs. Iron content of the olfactory bulb was increased ($p = 0.043$) in ID pigs compared with CONT pigs. Note that as iron content increases, quantitative susceptibility measures values change from diamagnetic (negative values) to paramagnetic (positive values). Abbreviations: control (CONT); iron deficient (ID). * Main effect of early-life dietary iron status, differs by $p < 0.05$.

Table 1. Quantitative susceptibility measures indicating iron concentrations (ppb) in defined brain regions of pigs differing in early-life iron status [1].

Region of interest	CONT		ID		SEM	Diet	Day	Diet × Day
	PND 32	PND 61	PND 32	PND 61				
Caudate	−6.3	−3.4	−2.1	−2.4	1.51	0.103	0.318	0.217
Cerebellum	4.6	1.6	0.9	0.5	0.91	0.005	0.069	0.144
Cerebral Aqueduct	−9.0	−15.8	−13.3	−9.2	3.14	0.723	0.609	0.065
Corpus Callosum	0.6	5.3	−0.1	4.5	2.04	0.676	0.029	0.994
Fourth Ventricle	−1.1	−9.8	−3.6	−7.5	3.59	0.985	0.057	0.428
Hypothalamus	−4.7	−11.0	−2.6	−6.3	2.48	0.161	0.044	0.550
Internal Capsule	−8.6	−8.0	−9.5	−7.5	1.04	0.760	0.303	0.560
Lateral Ventricle	−3.8	−1.3	−4.3	−2.4	1.48	0.542	0.110	0.834
Left Cortex	−0.6	−0.5	−2.2	−2.8	0.60	0.004	0.614	0.470
Left Hippocampus	−0.5	−1.9	−7.6	−6.9	1.53	<0.001	0.811	0.447
Medulla	5.1	5.3	−0.2	1.5	2.09	0.018	0.666	0.729
Midbrain	−6.5	−6.0	−8.8	−7.8	2.15	0.351	0.684	0.867
Olfactory Bulb	0.4	−0.2	1.6	1.5	0.77	0.043	0.601	0.715
Pons	4.7	10.9	−6.5	−2.2	2.83	<0.001	0.064	0.702
Putamen-Globus Pallidus	−6.3	−3.9	−5.1	−4.5	1.22	0.786	0.175	0.392
Right Cortex	−1.0	0.0	−2.7	−0.5	0.72	0.083	0.033	0.383
Right Hippocampus	−3.2	−0.6	−7.0	−4.2	2.29	0.141	0.127	0.979
Thalamus	−7.7	−11.0	−7.0	−7.6	1.88	0.322	0.166	0.319
Third Ventricle	−4.1	−4.8	−1.8	0.9	2.49	0.105	0.663	0.433

[1] Data presented as least square means and pooled standard errors of the mean (SEM) for each treatment group. Statistical significance of the main effects of early-life dietary treatment (Diet; CONT vs. ID) and postnatal magnetic resonance imaging (MRI) day (Day; PND 32 vs. 61) and the interaction between Diet and Day are presented. Number of pigs per treatment group that were subjected to MRI are as follows: PND 32 (CONT, *n* = 9–11; ID, *n* = 8–10), PND 61 (CONT, *n* = 5–7; ID, *n* = 7–9). In general susceptibility measures increase from negative (diamagnetic) to positive (paramagnetic) as iron accumulates in tissues. Abbreviations: control (CONT), iron deficient (ID), parts per billion (ppb), postnatal day (PND).

3.2. Voxel-Based Morphometry

Voxel-based morphometry is an analytical technique used to compare grey or white matter tissue distribution between two treatment groups. Accordingly, each treatment group may have more or less grey matter or white matter, resulting in clusters of voxels that indicate differences in tissue composition. Analysis of grey and white matter tissue segmentations from the PND 61 imaging time-point indicated region-specific differences ($p < 0.001$) between CONT and ID pigs, Table 2. A comparison of grey matter voxels where CONT pigs exhibited more ($p < 0.001$) grey matter voxels than ID pigs indicated differences in the left cortex, right cortex, cerebellum, hippocampus, thalamus, and caudate (CONT > ID), Figure 2 (red comparisons). The opposite comparison, in which ID pigs exhibited increased grey matter ($p < 0.001$) compared with CONT pigs (ID > CONT) indicated small grey matter clusters, in each of the left and right cortex, Figure 2 (blue comparisons). Comparison of white matter voxels where CONT pigs exhibited more ($p < 0.001$) white matter voxels than ID pigs indicated differences in the internal capsule, left cortex, right cortex, left hippocampus, and right hippocampus (CONT > ID), Figure 3 (red comparisons) and Table 2. There were no instances in which ID pigs exhibited more white matter compared with CONT pigs (ID > CONT). Table 2 lists clusters of edge-connected voxels where a statistical difference between the two dietary treatments was observed. The anatomical regions described were determined from *X*, *Y*, *Z* coordinates that corresponded to peak maximum differences within the clusters, thus it is possible to have multiple peaks per cluster.

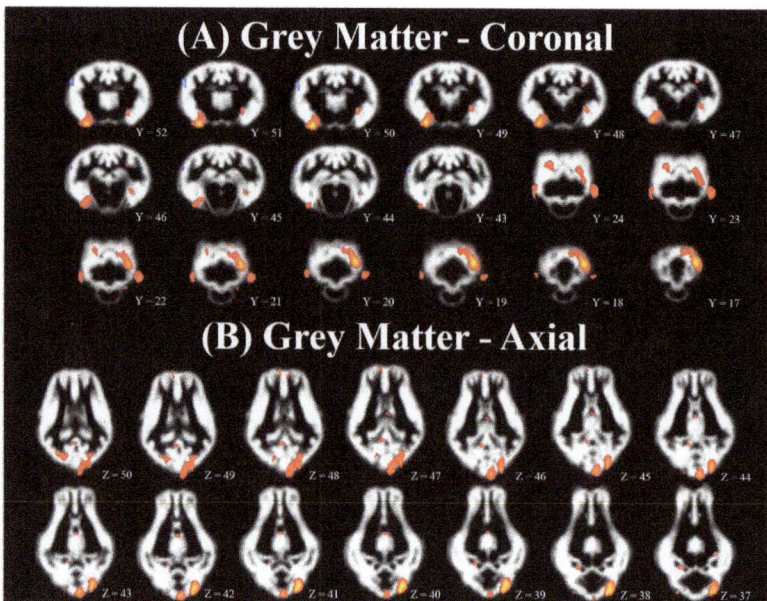

Figure 2. Pictured here is a population-averaged pig brain, with a statistical heat map indicating differences in grey matter between dietary treatment groups. The range of red-to-yellow indicates the degree of statistical difference from significant pseudo-*t* values of 3.80 to 7.35, respectively, in voxels where CONT pigs exhibited increased grey matter concentrations compared with ID pigs (i.e., CONT grey matter > ID grey matter). Clusters that range from dark-to-light blue indicate increasing significance from significant pseudo-*t* values of 4.30 to 5.55, respectively, in voxels where ID pigs exhibit increased grey matter compared with CONT pigs (i.e., ID grey matter > CONT grey matter). (**A**) Brain images in coronal orientation and (**B**) Brain images in axial orientation. Abbreviations: control (CONT); iron deficient (ID).

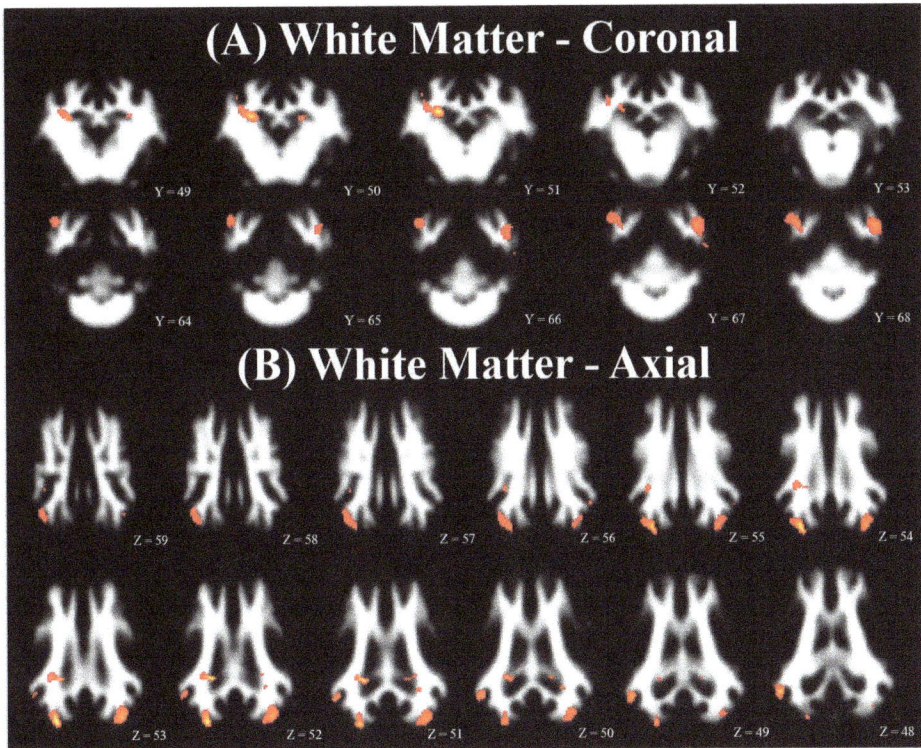

Figure 3. Pictured here is a population-averaged pig brain, with a statistical heat map indicating differences in white matter between dietary treatment groups. The range of red-to-yellow indicates the degree of statistical difference from significant pseudo-*t* values of 4.00 to 6.40, respectively, in voxels where CONT pigs exhibited increased white matter concentrations compared with ID pigs (i.e., CONT white matter > ID white matter). Notably, no differences were observed where ID pigs exhibited increased white matter concentrations compared with CONT pigs. (**A**) Brain images in coronal orientation and (**B**) Brain images in axial orientation. Abbreviations: control (CONT); iron deficient (ID).

3.3. Tract-Based Spatial Statistics

Tract-based spatial statistics allows assessment of differences due to diet in FA values along predetermined white matter tracts from data acquired at the PND 61 time-point. Analysis of FA values indicated subcortical areas in which CONT pigs exhibited greater ($p < 0.05$) FA values compared with ID pigs, Figure 4. Upon visual inspection, the greatest FA value differences appear to be in the white matter tracts located in the caudate and thalamus. Analysis of the opposite comparison, where FA values were greater in ID pigs compared with CONT pigs, revealed no differences ($p > 0.05$).

Table 2. Voxel-based morphometry assessment of grey and white matter at PND 61 comparing pigs from differing early-life iron status [1].

Tissue	Comparison	Anatomic Region [2]	Cluster Level Number of Voxels	Cluster Level p-Value	Peak Level p-Value	Peak Level Pseudo-t	X	Y	Z
		Right Cortex	2045	<0.001	<0.001	7.31	14.0	0.0	-12.6
		Right Cortex			<0.001	5.32	18.9	-13.3	-8.4
		Cerebellum	2772	<0.001	<0.001	6.92	-10.5	-25.2	0.0
		Cerebellum			<0.001	5.98	-2.8	-27.3	2.8
		Left Cortex			<0.001	5.16	-10.5	-16.8	5.6
		Right Cortex	443	0.004	<0.001	5.98	11.9	-15.4	7.7
		Cerebellum	997	<0.001	<0.001	5.55	-18.9	-18.9	-7.7
		Cerebellum	251	0.023	<0.001	5.54	9.1	-9.8	-2.1
Grey	CONT > ID	Right Hippocampus			<0.001	5.12	2.1	-9.1	6.3
		Left Cortex	242	0.025	<0.001	5.27	-14.0	-1.4	-3.5
		Left Cortex	204	0.037	<0.001	5.01	-13.3	-7.0	13.3
		Cerebellum	47	0.291	<0.001	4.83	11.9	-25.9	-2.8
		Thalamus	160	0.061	<0.001	4.36	0.0	10.5	0.7
		Right Cortex	79	0.175	<0.001	4.35	3.5	36.4	4.9
		Right Cortex	72	0.194	<0.001	4.15	13.3	-9.8	11.2
		Left Cortex	24	0.455	0.001	3.97	-5.6	-20.3	11.9
		Left Cortex	42	0.318	0.001	3.97	-2.1	33.6	5.6
		Caudate	21	0.486	0.001	3.81	2.1	18.2	2.8
		Right Cortex	419	0.005	<0.001	5.51	22.4	0.7	10.5
		Left Cortex	57	0.246	<0.001	4.45	-19.6	4.2	7.0
Grey	CONT <ID	Right Cortex	35	0.363	<0.001	4.34	18.2	16.1	12.6
		Right Hippocampus	234	0.022	<0.001	6.37	8.4	-2.1	8.4
		Right Cortex	629	0.001	<0.001	6.19	10.5	-16.8	9.1
		Right Cortex			<0.001	4.61	15.4	-9.8	13.3
		Right Cortex	378	0.005	<0.001	5.85	20.3	-7.0	4.2
		Left Cortex	653	0.001	<0.001	5.26	-14.0	-15.4	9.1
White	CONT > ID	Cerebellum			<0.001	4.26	-18.9	-16.1	0.7
		Internal Capsule	51	0.252	<0.001	4.48	-11.2	-5.6	7.7
		Left Hippocampus	61	0.212	<0.001	4.42	-7.0	-1.4	7.0
		Left Cortex	26	0.415	<0.001	4.07	-18.9	-7.7	11.2
		Internal Capsule	40	0.310	0.001	4.00	-8.4	20.3	3.5
White	CONT <ID	None	-	-	-	-	-	-	-

[1] Voxel-based morphometry analysis of gray and white matter differences in the CONT and ID pig brains at PND 61. A threshold of $p <0.001$ and minimum cluster size of 20 voxels were used to determine p-uncorrected values listed in the table. Abbreviations: control (CONT), iron deficient (ID). [2] Brain regions based on visual inspection of the cluster location and cross-referenced with the Piglet Brain Atlas [29]. [3] Local maxima coordinates: X increases from left (−) to right (+), Y increases from posterior (−) to anterior (+), and Z increases from inferior (−) to superior (+).

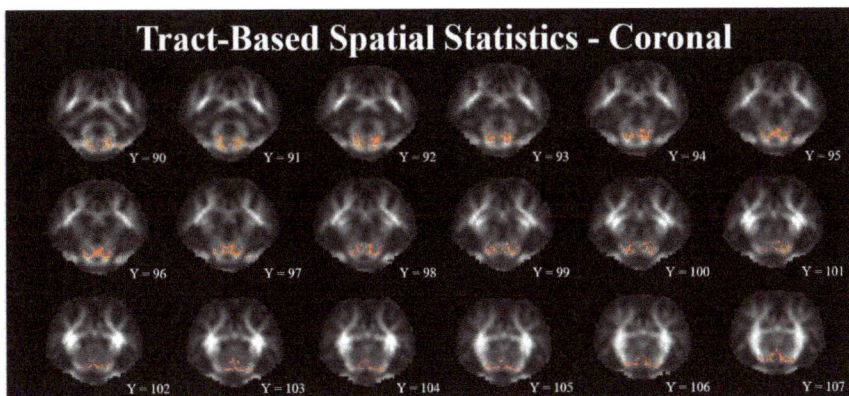

Figure 4. Pictured here is a population-averaged pig brain, with a statistical heat map indicating differences in white matter tract development between dietary treatment groups. Fractional anisotropy (FA) differences along predetermined white matter tracts where CONT pigs exhibited higher ($p < 0.05$) FA values compared with ID pigs. Representative slices were chosen to highlight areas in which FA values in CONT pigs were higher than in ID pigs. The range of red-to-yellow indicates degree of statistical difference from $p = 0.05$ to $p = 0.001$, respectively. Brain images in coronal orientation. Abbreviations: control (CONT); fractional anisotropy (FA); iron deficient (ID).

4. Discussion

Iron is pivotal for proper brain development, and alterations in both prenatal and postnatal iron status severely influence brain structure and function [4,6,16,36]. Moreover, brain development is a dynamic and heterogeneous process, thus the effects of iron deficiency are highly dependent on the timing and severity of the altered iron status [6]. In our study, pigs were provided either an ID or CONT diet from PND 2 until PND 32, at which point all pigs were switched to iron-replete diets until PND 61. The aim of this study was to determine what microstructural differences persisted in the brain at PND 61, despite all pigs being provided iron-replete diets from PND 33 to PND 61. In doing so, our study was designed to mimic postnatal dietary iron deficiency in human infants from birth up until four to six months of age when iron-fortified foods tend to be introduced into the diet. We previously published results indicating that total brain volumes are different between ID and CONT pigs at PND 32 but are not different at PND 61 [24]. Despite the observed compensatory brain volume growth during the period of dietary iron repletion, results from our analyses indicated tissue microstructural differences remained at PND 61. Therefore, to further elucidate how dietary iron status influenced brain development, we used voxel-based morphometry and tract-based spatial statistics to provide visual characterizations of neurodevelopment at PND 61. Herein we provide evidence that structural differences in grey and white matter are present in specific regions of the brain, even after 30 days of iron repletion. We also utilized quantitative susceptibility mapping to non-invasively characterize differences in brain iron content due to early-life dietary iron deficiency. These results are poised to have clinical relevance as we show neuroimaging can sensitively quantify differences in brain iron content due to dietary iron status.

4.1. Quantitative Susceptibility Measures

Iron is essential throughout early-life brain development to facilitate proper myelination [15], neurotransmitter synthesis [16,17], and neuron morphology [18,19]. Accordingly, the concentration of iron varies by brain region [37,38] and its presence is critical to ensure proper development throughout the brain. To date, many animal studies have focused on quantification of brain iron using invasive techniques to analyze samples of brain tissue [14,26,39]. Importantly, assessment of iron status through blood biomarkers is not always a reliable predictor of brain iron content. As evidence of this, a recent study where pigs were provided with ID diets early in life followed by iron replete diets indicated hematocrit and hemoglobin measures were not different between CONT and ID pigs at 12 weeks of age, but hippocampal iron content remained lower in ID pigs [26]. Provided the ethical limitations of collecting brain samples from human infants and the unreliable relationship between blood and brain iron concentrations, there is a need for a non-invasive assessment of brain iron content early in life. Quantitative susceptibility mapping is a non-invasive neuroimaging technique which can be used to sensitively characterize brain iron content [32]. This technique quantifies magnetic properties of tissue, and as iron is deposited into tissue, the tissue becomes increasingly paramagnetic. Thus, as development occurs and iron is accreted, it is expected that QSM values will increase (indicating stronger paramagnetic tissue properties). A previous report, where QSM methods were used in children, indicates that increased brain iron concentrations in the caudate related to increased spatial IQ [23]. Accordingly, this method may prove to be a sensitive non-invasive biomarker for quantifying brain iron content, and may help to explain differences in brain structural and functional development. To our knowledge, there do not appear to be any studies using QSM to determine the iron status of infant brains, however this method has been shown to sensitively characterize altered iron content in clinical cases of restless leg syndrome [21] and β-thalassemia [22].

In the present analysis, we used QSM to assess whether differences in brain iron could be detected non-invasively after a period of early-life iron deficiency. Our results indicate that pigs provided an early-life ID diet exhibited decreased brain iron concentrations in the cerebellum, pons, medulla, left cortex, and right cortex compared with CONT pigs at PND 32 and after receiving iron replete diets (i.e., at PND 61). Interestingly, ID pigs exhibited increased iron content in the olfactory bulb compared with CONT pigs. Previous analysis of brain volumes and diffusion tensor measures in this group of pigs indicated decreased relative brain volumes in the left hippocampus and the cerebellum of ID pigs [24]. Iron is needed for growth and expansion of neurons as well as dendrite morphogenesis in rodents [40] and pigs [41]. Thus, our QSM data may suggest a mechanism whereby decreased brain iron content attenuated neuron growth in the left hippocampus and cerebellum, thereby resulting in reduced relative volumes of these regions. The suggestion that iron is necessary for neuron growth is also supported by our findings of increased brain iron content in the olfactory bulbs of ID pigs and our previous report of increased relative volumes of the olfactory bulbs in ID pigs [24]. It remains to be elucidated why the olfactory bulb exhibits opposite growth trends during an ID state, however this finding of increased brain iron content in the olfactory bulb adds to evidence that this is likely not a spurious finding. We previously reported decreased FA values in the left cortex and the cerebellum of ID pigs. Fractional anisotropy is often used as a non-invasive marker of myelination and fiber coherence in the brain and increases throughout development [42,43]. It is also known that iron is an essential co-factor in myelinating events [15,44,45]. Thus, the decreased iron concentrations in the cerebellum and left cortex further support our hypothesis of decreased myelination in these two brain regions in young pigs.

Interestingly, a study of brain iron content in adults ranging from 22 to 78 years of age indicated increased iron content in left hemisphere brain regions compared with right hemisphere regions [46]. Xu and colleagues [46] suggest that this hemispheric difference in iron content may be due to lateralization of motor control, which is largely controlled by the dopaminergic system and is dependent on iron for neurotransmitter synthesis. Although handedness in our pigs was not assessed, our data of decreased iron in the left hippocampus and left cortex in ID pigs compared with CONT pigs may suggest an apparent hemispheric sensitivity of brain iron accumulation due to dietary iron status. In a rodent model of chronic early-life iron deficiency followed by iron repletion into adulthood, concentrations of brain iron restored to levels not different than in CONT animals in all regions except the thalamus [17]. Results from our study assessed brain iron at PND 32 and 61 and only a main effect of dietary treatment was noted for the brain regions discussed. Thus, future research should seek to non-invasively characterize brain iron content after a longer period of repletion to identify if iron content in ID pig brains is able to recover to levels observed in CONT pigs. In doing so, researchers will be able to better define the extent of dietary iron adequacy that is necessary to restore brain iron content back to baseline levels within an individual. It should be noted, however, that Felt and colleagues [17] observed altered monoamine metabolism and behavior in adult rodents that were previously ID, indicating that restoring brain iron to normal levels may not be sufficient to counteract the alterations in brain development due to early life iron deficiency. Our QSM findings of altered brain iron content stand to have clinical relevance, as we were able to use a non-invasive neuroimaging technique to sensitively quantify differences in brain iron content between ID and CONT pigs. Knowing that brain iron tends to decrease prior to hematological decreases in iron [5], neuroimaging of at-risk infants may help to identify and correct alterations in brain iron before overt signs of clinical iron deficiency are observed.

It is also worth mentioning that three brain regions indicated a change of iron content over time that was independent of dietary treatment. Notably, we observed an increase in QSM values in the corpus callosum and right cortex from PND 31 to PND 62, whereas a decrease in values was observed in the hypothalamus. Because these findings did not indicate sensitivity to dietary treatment, it suggests that these regions might be more resilient or less affected by alterations in dietary iron status when accumulating iron-containing compounds. We previously reported no differences due to dietary iron status in diffusion tensor fractional anisotropy, a measure indicating myelin and fiber tract development, in the corpus callosum [24]. Despite the lack of dietary effect in the corpus callosum FA values [24], we did observe an increase in corpus callosum FA values over time, which is consistent with the QSM values we report herein. Notably, our analysis of FA values in the right cortex did indicate a dietary effect [24], whereas our QSM values did not exhibit an effect of diet. This might suggest that the presence of iron-containing compounds is not solely responsible for changes in brain structure. As this is one of the first studies to assess QSM over time in early development, it is unclear if the decrease in hypothalamus values is of physiological relevance. Thus, future work should seek to better characterize changes in QSM across multiple time points to elucidate the trajectory of QSM changes from birth until adulthood. Doing so in the context of a longer period of iron deficiency might illuminate brain regions that are susceptible to alterations in QSM at different time points throughout the developmental process.

4.2. Voxel-Based Morphometry

We previously reported a reduction of approximately 10% in total brain volume at PND 32 in ID pigs compared with CONT pigs. However, after a period of dietary iron repletion from PND 33 to 61, brain volumes were not statistically different between early life ID and CONT pigs [24]. Despite this finding of similar brain volume, we observed microstructural differences in diffusion tensor measures between the two groups at PND 61, indicating that dietary iron repletion did not recover all aspects of brain development. Therefore, to further explore these microstructural differences we used voxel-based morphometry to visually assess differences in grey and white matter tissue concentrations that remained present at PND 61. Assessment of grey matter tissue differences between CONT and ID pigs indicated more voxels in which CONT pigs had greater concentrations of grey matter compared with ID pigs. Interestingly, these clusters of increased grey matter in CONT pigs were located in the left cortex, right cortex, cerebellum, thalamus, caudate, and right hippocampus. A previous study of iron deficiency in 30-day-old pigs indicated differences in cortical grey matter in CONT pigs compared with ID pigs [47]. In our study and the study by Leyshon and colleagues, the most abundant differences in grey matter appeared to be localized to cortical brain regions. However, the differences that were observed by Leyshon and colleagues between CONT and ID pigs at 30 d of age contained more voxels and larger clusters than what we observed in our pigs after a period of iron repletion on PND 61. Thus, it is possible that a period of iron repletion may be able to compensate for some alterations in tissue grey matter, yet it is clear that structural differences are present after 30 days of iron repletion.

In a rodent model of perinatal iron deficiency, ID rodents exhibited decreased branching complexity of cortical apical and basal dendrites, but no difference in dendrite length when compared with CONT rodents [19]. Pigs that were provided ID diets from birth until 4 weeks of life and iron replete diets from 4 until 12 weeks of life exhibited no difference in brain-derived neurotrophic factor (BDNF) expression in the prefrontal cortex [48]. In pigs, cortical brain tissue is just reaching its maximal growth rate at 4 weeks of age [49], corresponding to the age at which our study and the study by Nelissen and colleagues [48] switched ID pigs to iron replete diets. Thus, the lack of difference in BDNF in the prefrontal cortex of 12-week-old pigs and our observation of similar brain volumes at 8 weeks of age between ID and CONT pigs may suggest neuron outgrowth was not drastically influenced by early-life iron deficiency. However, the persistent differences in localized grey matter concentrations in the cortex may suggest altered neuron morphology, thus corroborating the findings by Greminger and colleagues [19]. The observed reductions in right hippocampal grey matter in ID pigs may also be a result of altered dendritic arborization, as this has previously been observed in ID hippocampal cell cultures from rodents [18]. These findings may suggest a non-invasive technique for characterizing altered cortical neuronal complexity in pigs that were ID early in life.

When assessing white matter, CONT pigs exhibited localized increases in both hippocampi, both cortices, the cerebellum, and the internal capsule when compared with ID pigs. In contrast, assessment of regions in which ID pigs exhibited increased white matter compared with CONT pigs yielded no significant results. This finding substantiates previous findings in 30-day-old pigs in which ID pigs did not have any voxels containing more white matter when compared with CONT pigs [47]. Together, these findings indicate that once detriments in white matter maturation have occurred early in life, recovery may not be possible, even after a subsequent period of dietary iron repletion. This observation of decreased white matter also aligns with our previous results of decreased FA values in the whole brain, cortex, cerebellum, and internal capsule due to early-life iron deficiency in pigs [24]. Previous research indicates reduced cerebellar myelination in rodents [45], thus suggesting that our observed reductions in cerebellar white matter may be due to reduced myelination. A previous study of 30-day-old ID pigs also indicated reduced white matter concentrations in the internal capsule [47]. It is known that the internal capsule and cerebellum are critical for coordinating motor skills and previous research in ID and ID anemic infants indicates delayed motor development [8], thus our findings of reduced white matter concentrations in these regions may indicate reductions in myelin development. While our study did not assess motor coordination or gait analysis in young pigs, future work should seek to assess the effect of early life iron on these measures. Provided there remain differences in both grey and white matter after a 30 day period of dietary iron repletion, future studies should seek to characterize if there is a period of iron repletion that is capable of rendering CONT and ID brains structurally similar.

4.3. Tract-Based Spatial Statistics

Tract-based spatial statistics allows for comparison of diffusion values along predetermined white matter tracts in the brain. Our previous diffusion tensor analysis indicated reductions in whole brain FA values in ID pigs, as well as FA reductions in the caudate, cerebellum, and internal capsule [24]. These previous observations were averaged over all white matter found in a defined brain region and were not specific to white matter tracts. Provided our previous results indicated differences in diffusion values that persisted at PND 61, we used TBSS to visualize white matter tracts where early-life ID pigs exhibited decreased FA values relative to CONT pigs. Assessment of white matter tracts in which CONT pigs exhibited voxels with higher FA values compared with ID pigs indicated differences located exclusively in subcortical brain regions. From our analysis, the regions in which FA values were greater in CONT pigs along white matter tracts appear to be localized to the internal capsule, thalamus, and hypothalamus. Importantly, there were no voxels along white matter tracts in which ID pigs exhibited increased FA values compared with CONT pigs, thereby suggesting that iron deficiency only causes detriments in white matter integrity and does not support white matter maturation. As described above, decreased white matter was observed in the internal capsule of ID pigs compared with CONT pigs. Thus, our VBM findings and the differences in TBSS in the internal capsule may suggest decreased myelin content of this brain region. Moreover, ID and ID anemic infants are known to have delayed motor development [8], and both the internal capsule and thalamus contain motor projections within the brain [50,51]. Previous research in rodents indicates the thalamus is susceptible to dietary iron deficiency, resulting in alterations in monoamine metabolism [4,16,17]. Additionally, increased thalamic axial, radial, and mean diffusivity values were observed in ID pigs at PND 29, suggesting altered myelination in this region [47]. Thus, our findings of altered white matter tracts in these two regions may suggest decreased internal capsule and thalamic myelination, thereby affirming a mechanism through which motor development is delayed in ID infants. It is interesting to note that these differences persist despite a subsequent period of iron repletion in pigs, thus indicating either the period for iron repletion was not long enough or it was applied too late in development to allow for recovery of microstructural changes due to early-life iron deficiency. Future research should seek to quantify myelin content in these brain regions at different time-points during and after iron deficiency to more definitively link iron status and myelination.

4.4. Limitations

While the results of this study are novel, we cannot definitively conclude that iron repletion after a period of early-life iron deficiency is incapable of compensating for developmental differences. Future research should seek to quantify different periods of dietary iron repletion as well as the timing of first providing an iron replete diet. In doing so, researchers will be able to better quantify critical windows during which iron influences particular aspects of brain development. Provided the results of our study, we suggest that early-life iron deficiency through PND 32 in the pig greatly alters myelinating events and may influence morphology of grey matter, but it does not appear to influence overall brain growth.

5. Conclusions

We previously showed that iron deficiency alters whole brain volumes at PND 32 but iron repletion was able to correct for observed differences by PND 61. Here we have shown that despite similar brain volumes, differences in grey matter and white matter, as well as decreased white matter tract integrity, remain at PND 61. Thus, while gross brain morphology appeared unaltered, microstructural detriments in brain development persisted in pigs exposed to early-life iron deficiency followed by a period of iron repletion. Our results also indicate region-specific reductions in brain iron concentrations of ID pigs, regardless of imaging time-point. Notably, characterization of altered brain iron and grey and white matter tissue concentrations were observed through non-invasive techniques, thereby providing clinically relevant methods to assess similar results in human infants. Thus, it is possible that neuroimaging may be used to comprehensively characterize altered brain iron status in infants at risk of iron deficiency, prior to the presence of overt symptoms of iron deficiency or iron deficiency anemia.

Acknowledgments: We would like to thank Brian Berg and Rosaline Waworuntu for their advice in study design. Additionally, we would like to thank Mead Johnson Nutrition for the dietary treatments used in this study. We would like to thank Kristen Karkiewicz and the rest of the Piglet Nutrition and Cognition Laboratory staff for day-to-day pig rearing. Lastly, we would like to thank Brad Sutton and the rest of the Beckman Imaging Center staff for their help in imaging acquisition and data analysis.

Author Contributions: A.T.M., J.E.F., L.C.K., and R.N.D. were involved in study design and implementation. All authors (A.T.M., J.E.F., L.C.K., F.L., Z.-P.L. and R.N.D.) were involved in data acquisition, analysis, and interpretation. All authors read and approved the final version of this manuscript.

Conflicts of Interest: The authors declare no conflict of interest.

References

1. World Health Organization. *Micronutrient Deficiencies—Iron Deficiency Anemia*; World Health Organization: Geneva, Switzerland, 2017.
2. World Health Organization. *Iron Deficiency Anaemia: Assessment, Prevention, and Control: A Guide for Programme Managers*; World Health Organization: Geneva, Switzerland, 2010.
3. McLean, E.; Cogswell, M.; Egli, I.; Wojdyla, D.; de Benoist, B. Worldwide prevalence of anaemia, WHO Vitamin and Mineral Nutrition Information System, 1993–2005. *Public Health Nutr.* **2009**, *12*, 444. [CrossRef] [PubMed]
4. Lozoff, B.; Georgieff, M.K. Iron deficiency and brain development. *Semin. Pediatr. Neurol.* **2006**, *13*, 158–165. [CrossRef] [PubMed]
5. Georgieff, M.K. Iron assessment to protect the developing brain. *Am. J. Clin. Nutr.* **2017**, *106*, 1588S–1593S. [CrossRef] [PubMed]
6. Georgieff, M.K. Nutrition and the developing brain: Nutrient priorities and measurement. *Am. J. Clin. Nutr.* **2007**, *85*, 614–620.
7. Radlowski, E.C.; Johnson, R.W. Perinatal iron deficiency and neurocognitive development. *Front. Hum. Neurosci.* **2013**, *7*, 1–11. [CrossRef] [PubMed]
8. Shafir, T.; Angulo-Barroso, R.; Jing, Y.; Angelilli, M.L.; Jacobson, S.W.; Lozoff, B. Iron deficiency and infant motor development. *Early Hum. Dev.* **2008**, *84*, 479–485. [CrossRef] [PubMed]
9. Congdon, E.L.; Westerlund, A.; Algarin, C.R.; Peirano, P.D.; Gregas, M.; Lozoff, B.; Nelson, C.A. Iron deficiency in infancy is associated with altered neural correlates of recognition memory at 10 years. *J. Pediatr.* **2012**, *160*, 1027–1033. [CrossRef] [PubMed]
10. Lukowski, A.F.; Koss, M.; Burden, M.J.; Jonides, J.; Nelson, C.A.; Kaciroti, N.; Jimenez, E.; Lozoff, B. Iron deficiency in infancy and neurocognitive functioning at 19 years: Evidence of long-term deficits in executive function and recognition memory. *Nutr. Neurosci.* **2010**, *13*, 54–70. [CrossRef] [PubMed]
11. Lozoff, B.; Smith, J.B.; Kaciroti, N.; Clark, K.M.; Guevara, S.; Jimenez, E. Functional significance of early-life iron deficiency: Outcomes at 25 years. *J. Pediatr.* **2013**, *163*, 1260–1266. [CrossRef] [PubMed]
12. Algarín, C.; Peirano, P.; Garrido, M.; Pizarro, F.; Lozoff, B. Iron deficiency anemia in infancy: Long-lasting effects on auditory and visual system functioning. *Pediatr. Res.* **2003**, *53*, 217–223. [CrossRef] [PubMed]
13. Otero, G.A.; Fernández, T.; Pliego-Rivero, F.B.; Mendieta, G.G. Iron therapy substantially restores qEEG maturational lag among iron-deficient anemic infants. *Nutr. Neurosci.* **2017**, 1–10. [CrossRef] [PubMed]
14. Bastian, T.W.; Santarriaga, S.; Nguyen, T.A.; Prohaska, J.R.; Georgieff, M.K.; Anderson, G.W. Fetal and neonatal iron deficiency but not copper deficiency increases vascular complexity in the developing rat brain. *Nutr. Neurosci.* **2015**, *18*, 365–375. [CrossRef] [PubMed]
15. Todorich, B.; Pasquini, J.M.; Garcia, C.I.; Paez, P.M.; Connor, J.R. Oligodendrocytes and myelination: The role of iron. *Glia* **2009**, *57*, 467–478. [CrossRef] [PubMed]
16. Lozoff, B.; Unger, E.; Connor, J.; Felt, B.; Georgieff, M. Early iron deficiency has brain and behavior effects consistent with dopaminergic function. *J. Nutr.* **2011**, *141*, 740–746. [CrossRef] [PubMed]
17. Felt, B.T.; Beard, J.L.; Schallert, T.; Shao, J.; Aldridge, J.W.; Connor, J.R.; Georgieff, M.K.; Lozoff, B. Persistent neurochemical and behavioral abnormalities in adulthood despite early iron supplementation for perinatal iron deficiency anemia in rats. *Behav. Brain Res.* **2006**, *171*, 261–270. [CrossRef] [PubMed]
18. Bastian, T.W.; Von Hohenberg, W.C.; Mickelson, D.J.; Lanier, L.M.; Georgieff, M.K. Iron deficiency impairs developing hippocampal neuron gene expression, energy metabolism, and dendrite complexity. *Dev. Neurosci.* **2016**, *38*, 264–276. [CrossRef] [PubMed]
19. Greminger, A.R.; Lee, D.L.; Shrager, P.; Mayer-Proschel, M. Gestational iron deficiency differentially alters the structure and function of white and gray matter brain regions of developing rats. *J. Nutr.* **2014**, *144*, 1058–1066. [CrossRef] [PubMed]
20. Monk, C.; Georgieff, M.K.; Xu, D.; Hao, X.; Bansal, R.; Gustafsson, H.; Spicer, J.; Peterson, B.S. Maternal prenatal iron status and tissue organization in the neonatal brain. *Pediatr. Res.* **2016**, *79*, 482–488. [CrossRef] [PubMed]
21. Li, X.; Allen, R.P.; Earley, C.J.; Liu, H.; Cruz, T.E.; Edden, R.A.E.; Barker, P.B.; van Zijl, P.C.M. Brain iron deficiency in idiopathic restless legs syndrome measured by quantitative magnetic susceptibility at 7 tesla. *Sleep Med.* **2016**, *22*, 75–82. [CrossRef] [PubMed]

22. Qiu, D.; Chan, G.C.-F.; Chu, J.; Chan, Q.; Ha, S.-Y.; Moseley, M.E.; Khong, P.-L. MR quantitative susceptibility imaging for the evaluation of iron loading in the brains of patients with β-thalassemia. *Am. J. Neuroradiol.* **2014**, *35*, 1085–1090. [CrossRef] [PubMed]

23. Carpenter, K.L.H.; Li, W.; Wei, H.; Wu, B.; Xiao, X.; Liu, C.; Worley, G.; Egger, H.L. Magnetic susceptibility of brain iron is associated with childhood spatial IQ. *Neuroimage* **2016**, *132*, 167–174. [CrossRef] [PubMed]

24. Mudd, A.; Fil, J.; Knight, L.; Dilger, R. Dietary iron repletion following early-life dietary iron deficiency does not correct regional volumetric or diffusion tensor changes in the developing pig brain. *Front. Neurol.* **2017**. [CrossRef]

25. Gan, L.; Yang, B.; Mei, H. The effect of iron dextran on the transcriptome of pig hippocampus. *Genes Genom.* **2017**, *39*, 1–14. [CrossRef]

26. Antonides, A.; Schoonderwoerd, A.C.; Scholz, G.; Berg, B.M.; Nordquist, R.E.; van der Staay, F.J. Pre-weaning dietary iron deficiency impairs spatial learning and memory in the cognitive holeboard task in piglets. *Front. Behav. Neurosci.* **2015**, *9*, 1–16. [CrossRef] [PubMed]

27. National Research Council (USA). *Nutrient Requirements of Swine*, 11th ed.; The National Academies Press: Washington, DC, USA, 2012.

28. Mudd, A.T.; Getty, C.; Sutton, B.; Dilger, R. Perinatal choline deficiency delays brain development and alters metabolite concentrations in the young pig. *Nutr. Neurosci.* **2016**, *19*, 425–433. [CrossRef] [PubMed]

29. Conrad, M.S.; Sutton, B.P.; Dilger, R.N.; Johnson, R. An in vivo three-dimensional magnetic resonance imaging-based averaged brain collection of the neonatal piglet (Sus scrofa). *PLoS ONE* **2014**, *9*, 107650. [CrossRef] [PubMed]

30. Lam, F.; Liang, Z.-P. A subspace approach to high-resolution spectroscopic imaging. *Magn. Reson. Med.* **2014**, *71*, 1349–1357. [CrossRef] [PubMed]

31. Peng, X.; Lam, F.; Li, Y.; Clifford, B.; Liang, Z.-P. Simultaneous QSM and metabolic imaging of the brain using SPICE. *Magn. Reson. Med.* **2018**, *79*, 13–21. [CrossRef] [PubMed]

32. Wang, Y.; Liu, T. Quantitative susceptibility mapping (QSM): Decoding MRI data for a tissue magnetic biomarker. *Magn. Reson. Med.* **2015**, *73*, 82–101. [CrossRef] [PubMed]

33. Zhou, D.; Liu, T.; Spincemaille, P.; Wang, Y. Background field removal by solving the Laplacian boundary value problem. *NMR Biomed.* **2014**, *27*, 312–319. [CrossRef] [PubMed]

34. Smith, S.M.; Jenkinson, M.; Woolrich, M.W.; Beckmann, C.F.; Behrens, T.E.J.; Johansen-Berg, H.; Bannister, P.R.; De Luca, M.; Drobnjak, I.; Flitney, D.E.; et al. Advances in functional and structural MR image analysis and implementation as FSL. *Neuroimage* **2004**, *23*, S208–S219. [CrossRef] [PubMed]

35. Smith, S.M.; Jenkinson, M.; Johansen-Berg, H.; Rueckert, D.; Nichols, T.E.; Mackay, C.E.; Watkins, K.E.; Ciccarelli, O.; Cader, M.Z.; Matthews, P.M.; et al. Tract-based spatial statistics: Voxelwise analysis of multi-subject diffusion data. *Neuroimage* **2006**, *31*, 1487–1505. [CrossRef] [PubMed]

36. Georgieff, M.K. Long-term brain and behavioral consequences of early iron deficiency. *Nutr. Rev.* **2011**, *69*, 43–48. [CrossRef] [PubMed]

37. Haacke, E.M.; Cheng, N.Y.C.; House, M.J.; Liu, Q.; Neelavalli, J.; Ogg, R.J.; Khan, A.; Ayaz, M.; Kirsch, W.; Obenaus, A. Imaging iron stores in the brain using magnetic resonance imaging. *Magn. Reson. Imaging* **2005**, *23*, 1–25. [CrossRef] [PubMed]

38. Bradbury, M.W. Transport of iron in the blood-brain-cerebrospinal fluid system. *J. Neurochem.* **1997**, *69*, 443–454. [CrossRef] [PubMed]

39. Rytych, J.L.; Elmore, M.R.P.; Burton, M.D.; Conrad, M.S.; Donovan, S.M.; Dilger, R.N.; Johnson, R.W. Early life iron deficiency impairs spatial cognition in neonatal piglets. *J. Nutr.* **2012**, *142*, 2050–2056. [CrossRef] [PubMed]

40. Jorgenson, L.A.; Wobken, J.D.; Georgieff, M.K. Perinatal iron deficiency alters apical dendritic growth in hippocampal CA1 pyramidal neurons. *Dev. Neurosci.* **2003**, *25*, 412–420. [CrossRef] [PubMed]

41. Schachtschneider, K.M.; Liu, Y.; Rund, L.A.; Madsen, O.; Johnson, R.W.; Groenen, M.A.M.; Schook, L.B. Impact of neonatal iron deficiency on hippocampal DNA methylation and gene transcription in a porcine biomedical model of cognitive development. *BMC Genom.* **2016**, *17*, 856. [CrossRef] [PubMed]

42. Drobyshevsky, A.; Song, S.; Gamkrelidze, G.; Wyrwicz, A.M.; Derrick, M.; Meng, F.; Li, L.; Ji, X.; Trommer, B.; Beardsley, D.J.; et al. Developmental changes in diffusion anisotropy coincide with immature oligodendrocyte progression and maturation of compound action potential. *J. Neurosci.* **2005**, *25*, 5988–5997. [CrossRef] [PubMed]

43. Hermoye, L.; Saint-Martin, C.; Cosnard, G.; Lee, S.-K.; Kim, J.; Nassogne, M.-C.; Menten, R.; Clapuyt, P.; Donohue, P.K.; Hua, K.; et al. Pediatric diffusion tensor imaging: Normal database and observation of the white matter maturation in early childhood. *Neuroimage* **2006**, *29*, 493–504. [CrossRef] [PubMed]

44. Wu, L.-L.; Zhang, L.; Shao, J.; Qin, Y.-F.; Yang, R.-W.; Zhao, Z.-Y. Effect of perinatal iron deficiency on myelination and associated behaviors in rat pups. *Behav. Brain Res.* **2008**, *188*, 263–270. [CrossRef] [PubMed]

45. Yu, G.S.; Steinkirchner, T.M.; Rao, G.A.; Larkin, E.C. Effect of prenatal iron deficiency on myelination in rat pups. *Am. J. Pathol.* **1986**, *125*, 620–624. [PubMed]

46. Xu, X.; Wang, Q.; Zhang, M. Age, gender, and hemispheric differences in iron deposition in the human brain: An in vivo MRI study. *Neuroimage* **2008**, *40*, 35–42. [CrossRef] [PubMed]

47. Leyshon, B.J.; Radlowski, E.C.; Mudd, A.T.; Steelman, A.J.; Johnson, R.W. Postnatal iron deficiency impairs brain development in piglets. *J. Nutr.* **2016**, *146*, 1420–1427. [CrossRef] [PubMed]

48. Nelissen, E.; De Vry, J.; Antonides, A.; Paes, D.; Schepers, M.; van der Staay, F.J.; Prickaerts, J.; Vanmierlo, T. Early-postnatal iron deficiency impacts plasticity in the dorsal and ventral hippocampus in piglets. *Int. J. Dev. Neurosci.* **2017**, *59*, 47–51. [CrossRef] [PubMed]

49. Conrad, M.S.; Dilger, R.N.; Johnson, R.W. Brain growth of the domestic pig (Sus scrofa) from 2 to 24 weeks of age: A longitudinal MRI study. *Dev. Neurosci.* **2012**, *34*, 291–298. [CrossRef] [PubMed]

50. Rose, J.; Mirmiran, M.; Butler, E.E.; Lin, C.Y.; Barnes, P.D.; Kermoian, R.; Stevenson, D.K. Neonatal microstructural development of the internal capsule on diffusion tensor imaging correlates with severity of gait and motor deficits. *Dev. Med. Child Neurol.* **2007**, *49*, 745–750. [CrossRef] [PubMed]

51. Hartmann-von Monakow, K.; Akert, K.; Künzle, H. Projections of the precentral motor cortex and other cortical areas of the frontal lobe to the subthalamic nucleus in the monkey. *Exp. Brain Res.* **1978**, *33*, 395–403. [CrossRef]

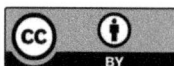

© 2018 by the authors. Licensee MDPI, Basel, Switzerland. This article is an open access article distributed under the terms and conditions of the Creative Commons Attribution (CC BY) license (http://creativecommons.org/licenses/by/4.0/).

nutrients

MDPI

Article

Chronic Monosodium Glutamate Administration Induced Hyperalgesia in Mice

Anca Zanfirescu, Aurelia Nicoleta Cristea [†], George Mihai Nitulescu *, Bruno Stefan Velescu and Daniela Gradinaru

Faculty of Pharmacy, "Carol Davila" University of Medicine and Pharmacy, TraianVuia 6, 020956 Bucharest, Romania; zanfirescuanca@yahoo.com (A.Z.); anicoletacristea@yahoo.com (A.N.C); bruno_velescu@yahoo.co.uk (B.S.V.); danielagrdnr@yahoo.com (D.G.)

*   Correspondence: nitulescu_mihai@yahoo.com; Tel.: +40-021-318-0739; Fax: +40-021-318-0750

†   In Memoriam: The authors would like to respectfully dedicate this article to Prof. Aurelia Nicoleta Cristea who passed away on 24 November 2017.

Received: 27 September 2017; Accepted: 14 December 2017; Published: 21 December 2017

Abstract: Monosodium glutamate (MSG) is a widely used food additive. Although it is generally considered safe, some questions regarding the impact of its use on general health have arisen. Several reports correlate MSG consumption with a series of unwanted reactions, including headaches and mechanical sensitivity in pericranial muscles. Endogenous glutamate plays a significant role in nociceptive processing, this neurotransmitter being associated with hyperalgesia and central sensitization. One of the mechanisms underlying these phenomena is the stimulation of Ca^{2+}/calmodulin sensitive nitric oxide synthase, and a subsequent increase in nitric oxide production. This molecule is a key player in nociceptive processing, with implications in acute and chronic pain states. Our purpose was to investigate the effect of this food additive on the nociceptive threshold when given orally to mice. Hot-plate and formalin tests were used to assess nociceptive behaviour. We also tried to determine if a correlation between chronic administration of MSG and variations in central nitric oxide (NO) concentration could be established. We found that a dose of 300 mg/kg MSG given for 21 days reduces the pain threshold and is associated with a significant increase in brain NO level. The implications of these findings on food additive-drug interaction, and on pain perception in healthy humans, as well as in those suffering from affections involving chronic pain, are still to be investigated.

Keywords: monosodium glutamate; hyperalgesia; hot-plate test; formalin test; nitric oxide synthase

1. Introduction

Monosodium glutamate (MSG), the salt of glutamic acid, is widely used as a food additive (E621). Two enantiomers are known, but only the naturally occurring isomer *L* is used as a flavor enhancer. Kwok, in 1968 [1], reported transient subjective symptoms (flushing, headache, numbness, general weakness, palpitation) following consumption of Chinese dishes known to contain high concentrations of E621. Several human studies were conducted afterwards to determine if a causal relationship existed between MSG and this symptom complex, but the results were inconsistent. The Joint FAO/WHO Expert Committee on Food Additives in 1971 [2], 1974 [3], and 1987 allocated it an "acceptable daily intake (ADI) not specified", considering MSG consumption to be safe [4]. The total intake of glutamate from food in European countries was assessed to range between 5 and 12 g/day, taking into account both natural and added glutamate [5].

Although MSG consumption is believed to be safe, several reports correlate MSG consumption with a series of unwanted reactions, including headache and mechanical sensitivity in pericranial muscles [5,6]. Clinical reports state that MSG consumption increases the frequency of fibromyalgia symptoms [7].

L-glutamate is a fast excitatory neurotransmitter with a significant role in nociceptive processing [8]. Two types of glutamate receptors are currently known: ligand-gated ion channels (NMDA, AMPA, kainate), and G protein-coupled receptors (metabotropic receptors) [9]. These receptors are well expressed in the central and peripheral nervous system, and have a high distribution in pain pathways [10–12]. Intraperitoneal or intrathecal administration of glutamate or agonists selective for one type of glutamate receptor induces nociceptive behaviors. Treatments with NMDA and AMPA antagonists or with inhibitors of glutamate release significantly reduce the hyperalgesia induced in experimental rodent models of acute inflammatory and neuropathic pain [13,14].

One of the mechanisms linked with NMDA-mediated hyperalgesia is stimulation of Ca^{2+}/calmodulin sensitive nitric oxide synthase, and a subsequent increase in nitric oxide (NO) production [15]. This molecule is a key player in nociceptive processing, with implications in acute [16] and chronic pain states [13]. The peripheral and central (mostly spinal) role of NO in nociceptive response was investigated in different animal models. Rat response to mechanical stimuli in a paradoxical sleep deprivation hyperalgesia model has been associated to nitric oxide synthase (NOS) activity enhancement in dorsolateral grey matter, leading to changes in the descendent modulating pain pathways [17]. Knock-out mice, lacking NOS encoding genes, showed a decrease of the tactile allodyniain mechanical stimulus test [18]. Nx-nitro-L-arginine methyl ester (L-NAME), a non-selective NOS inhibitor reduced the behavioral signs of neuropathic pain induced in rats by constricting the spinal [19] and sciatic [20] nerves. Intrathecal administration of L-NAME or of methylene blue, a soluble guanylatecyclase inhibitor, suppresses the thermal hyperalgesia induced in the sciatic nerve constriction model. Pretreatment with NOS inhibitors significantly attenuated the thermal hyperalgesia induced by the intraplantar injection of complete Freund's adjuvant in mice [21].

Taking into account the involvement of endogenous glutamate in pain processing and the different existing reports on MSG, we hypothesized that oral administration of this flavor enhancer would modify the nociceptive threshold when orally administered in mice. We also tried to determine some of the molecular changes underlying this effect.

2. Materials and Methods

2.1. Chemicals

Drugs and reagents employed were as follows: L-glutamic acid monosodium salt monohydrate, L-arginine, formaldehyde solution for molecular biology (36.5–38% in water), phosphate-buffered saline (PBS), Folin & Ciocalteu's phenol reagent, N-(1-naphthyl)-ethylenediaminedihydrochloride, cadmium chloride. All reagents were purchased from Sigma-Aldrich (St. Louis, MO, USA).

2.2. Animals

All experiments were performed in 5 weeks male NMRI mice (n = 60; 30 ± 3.6 g), purchased from UMF Biobase (Bucharest, Romania). They were housed 10 animals per cage (35.5 cm × 22.9 cm × 15.2 cm), in a ventilated cage system, with a bedding of wood sawdust, under controlled light/dark cycle conditions (12 h light/12 h dark; lights on at 6:00 a.m.), with free access to water and food pellets. The temperature ranged between 20 and 22 °C, and the relative humidity was maintained at 35–45%. All reagents were purchased from Sigma-Aldrich (St. Louis, MO, USA). All procedures were carried out according to EU Directive 2010/63/UE, and with the approval of the Institutional Animal Care and Use Committee. The study was approved by the Bioethics Commission of the University of Medicine and Pharmacy Bucharest with the ethical approval code 589/04.09.2016. For each experiment we used 30 mice, divided in three equal groups. The animals received the test solutions for 21 days by means of a straight animal ball-tipped feeding needle. The body weight evolution was constant during the experiment for all three groups, exhibiting no significant differences. After 21 days the mice body weight was 41 ± 4 g.

2.3. Formalin-Induced Nociception

Group I represented the control, and was given distilled water 1 mL/100 g, group II received 150 mg/kg MSG (1.5% MSG solution), and group III 300 mg/kg MSG (3.0% MSG solution). All solutions were prepared in distilled water. The doses of MSG used were selected following multiple tests, as reported previously [22]. Mice were injected with 20 μL of formalin reagent containing formaldehyde 1.2% in PBS into the plantar surface of the left hind-paw with a 30-gauge needle. They were then placed in a Plexiglas box (30 cm × 30 cm × 30 cm) with a mirror below the floor at a 45 degree angle to allow an unobstructed view of the paws. The total time spent by animal either licking or biting the injected paw (reaction time) was recorded for the following 50 min. We took into account the biphasic behavior induced by formalin: an initial acute phase (with a duration of 0–5 min, neurogenic pain), followed by a prolonged tonic response (between 25 and 50 min, inflammatory pain). Between phases 1 and 2, there was an intermittent period where little nociceptive behavior was observed. The total time spent by animal licking or biting the paw injected with formalin was considered an index of nociception in the formalin test.

2.4. Hot-Plate Latency Assay

Groups of ten mice received doses of 150 and 300 mg/kg MSG orally for 21 days, while the control group was administered with the vehicle. On day 21, animals were treated and brought into the testing room one hour before testing. Animals were placed in the testing chamber and allowed to acclimate for 1 h. For testing, mice were put into a fiberglass cylinder (15 cm diameter, 30 cm high) on a metal base, maintained at a temperature of $53 \pm 1\,°C$. Paw withdrawal latency to thermal noxious stimuli and latency of jumping response were used to assess the effects of substances on the thermal nociceptive threshold (Hot Plate, UgoBasile, Italy). In the absence of a response, the cut-off time was set to 45 s to prevent extensive damage of tissue. Hind-paw lifting was defined as lifting a hind-paw completely off the hot-plate. After 2 h, animals were sacrificed by decapitation, and the brain was harvested on ice. The biological material was used for the biochemical assays.

2.5. Assay of NO-Synthase (NOS) Activity

Total NOS activity was determined in crude tissue homogenates using the Griess method for human plasma adapted for brain tissue [23]. Using this method, we determined the concentration of NO metabolites: nitrites and nitrates (NOx). Freshly harvested brains were homogenized with PBS 1:5, centrifuged $10\times$ *g* min/2000 rpm and the supernatant further used. The brains were homogenized, centrifuged and then kept on ice until all culls were complete. Cofactors and substrate were added according to Table 1.

Table 1. Working method for NO metabolites (NOx) determination.

Reagents (μL)	Test	Control
Supernatant	360	360
PBS	310	540
L-Arginine [1]	60	-
FAD [2]	60	-
NADPH [3]	10	-
37 °C, 60 min		
Cadmium chloride	0.5 g/mL	0.5 g/mL
25 °C, 30 min		
Griess reagent	1000	1000

[1] 1.3 mg L-arginine/10 mL solution; [2] 0.6 mg FAD/10 mL solution; [3] 12.5 mg NADPH/1 mL solution. PBS, phosphate-buffered saline.

The reagents were stored on ice. Between each addition of cofactor/substrate, the aliquots were vortexed. The cofactors/substrates were prepared in PBS. When left for 60 or 30 min, the aliquots were left on a rocker. The nitrates were reduced to nitrites in the presence of cadmium, and treated with a diazotizing reagent, sulfanilamide, in acidic media to form a transient diazonium salt. This intermediate reacts with the coupling reagent, N-(1-naphthyl)-ethylenediaminedihydrochloride, to form a stable azo compound. The intense purple color of the product allows nitrite assay with high sensitivity, which was used to measure nitrite concentration spectrophotometrically at 660 nm (Chemwell2010, Awareness Technology, Inc., Palm City, FL, USA).

2.6. Total Protein Assay

The total protein concentration for the same samples of brain tissue was determined using the Lowry protein assay [24]. Diluted protein solutions treated with copper salts in basic pH and Folin & Ciocalteu's phenol reagent (hexavalent phosphomolybdic/phosphotungstic acid complexes) lead to the formation of blue compounds, whose concentration is linearly proportional to the protein concentration in the sample. NOx concentration was expressed for 1mg of protein.

2.7. Statistical Analysis

Statistical analysis was performed using GraphPad Prism version 5.00 for Windows, (GraphPad Software, San Diego, CA, USA). The type of distribution of the animal response was established with D'Agostino & Pearson test. Data are reported as means $\pm$ standard error of the mean (SEM), and were analyzed statistically using parametrical Student's t-Test, a confidence interval (CI) of 90%, and with p values of 0.05 or less being considered to be significant.

3. Results

3.1. Formalin-Induced Nociception

The control group exhibited a typical biphasic nociceptive response: increased time of reaction in the first 5 min, a reduction in response for approximately 10 min, and a subsequent increased level of nociceptive response, which began 15 min after formalin injection, and lasted until the end of the experiment. The results (Figure 1) showed that, in the first phase of the formalin test, there were no significant differences between the tested groups, although a slight increase in reaction time (7.05%) was noticed for group III-MSG 300 mg/kg vs. control.

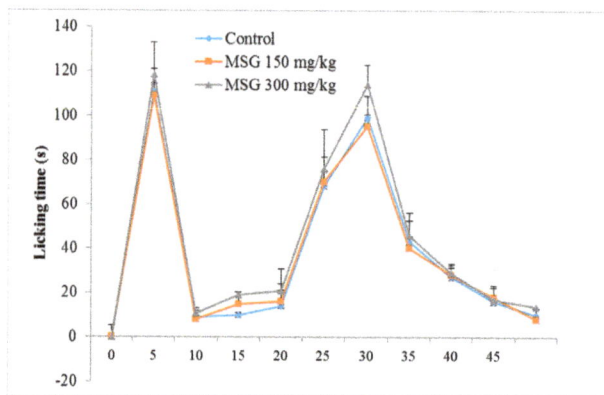

Figure 1. Time course of the formalin test in control (—◆—) and in Monosodium glutamate (MSG) treated mice (—■— MSG 150mg/kg; —▲— MSG 300 mg/kg). Values represent means $\pm$ standard error of the mean (SEM) of 10 animals.

For phase 2, characterized by inflammatory pain, MSG administered in a dose of 300 mg/kg determined a significant increase in the mean reaction time vs. the control group (11.31%, $p < 0.05$). In addition, the frequency of nociceptive responses during the normally quiet intermediate phase was similar to that of the late phase of the formalin test.

3.2. Hot-Plate Latency Assay

We tested the effects of oral dosing of MSG on baseline heat pain thresholds in mice. Previous studies showed no significant changes vs. the control group in hot-plate assay after seven days of MSG oral administration, for either 150 mg/kg or 300 mg/kg dosage. Only a slight, non-significant, reduction of the pain threshold was seen, after 14 days of MSG 300 mg/kg administration (data not published). Oral administration of MSG in doses of 150 mg/kg and 300 mg/kg significantly reduced the average latency of hind-paw lifting vs. baseline (−29.69% and −40.43%, respectively, all $p < 0.05$), following 21 days of administration. However, only the dose of 300 mg/kg MSG significantly reduced (−30.03%, $p < 0.05$) the average latency of hind-paw lifting vs. control (Figure 2). For the latency of jumping time, a significantly larger number of animals jumped when compared to the control group (data not shown).

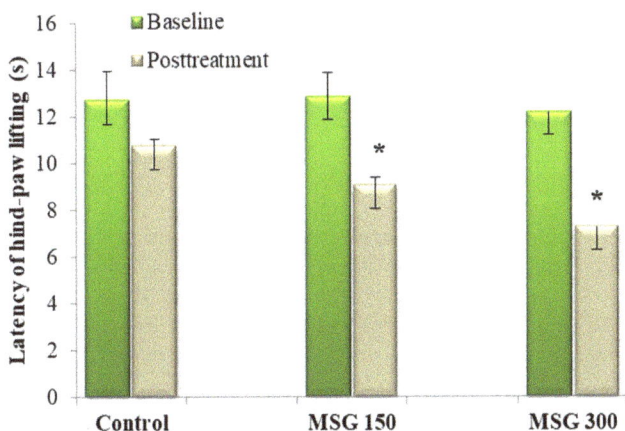

Figure 2. Medium latency of hind-paw lifting ± SEM before and after 21 days of MSG exposure. * Statistical significance vs. baseline (Student's *t*-Test, 90% CI, $p < 0.05$) and control group (Student's *t*-Test, 90% CI, $p < 0.05$).

3.3. Assay of NO-Synthase (NOS) Activity

NOS activity was assessed indirectly, by determining the concentration of NO metabolites (NOx). Administration of 300 mg/kg MSG for 21 days determined an increase of NOx concentration in the brain, and therefore an intensification of NOS activity in brain tissue (Figure 3). There were no changes in the total concentration of brain proteins when compared with the control.

We established a direct correlation between the increase in NOx concentration and the hyperalgic response to repeated administration of MSG (Spearman correlation, $p < 0.05$). Further studies will establish the effect of MSG administration on NOx in nociceptive behavior-naïve mice.

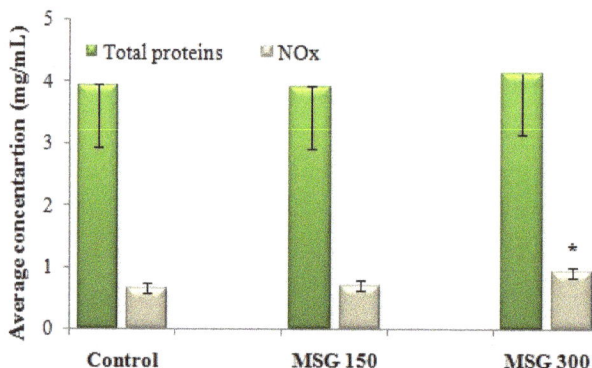

Figure 3. Average concentration of NO metabolites (NOx) in brain tissue after 21 days of exposure to distilled water (control) or MSG (150 mg/kg or 300 mg/kg). NOx concentration, as determined with the Griess method (x), is reported against the total protein concentration assessed in the same sample of brain tissue (y). The NOx concentration per 1 mg of protein = x/y. * Statistical significance vs. control (Student's t-Test, 90% CI, $p < 0.05$).

4. Discussion

Administration of MSG in a dosage of 300 mg/kg reduces the thermal nociceptive threshold and increases nociceptive behavior. The effect of MSG on the thermal threshold was correlated with an increase in NOx concentration, which suggests that the hyperalgic effect of MSG could be mediated via this messenger.

There is no literature data on the effect of MSG oral administration on the thermal threshold, as far as we know. Hot-plate is an objective, quantifiable, specific central antinociceptive test used to study the response to a noxious thermal stimulus [25,26]. The involvement of nitric oxide in nociceptive processing is generally recognized, with this molecule playing a pivotal role in hyperalgesia and central sensitization [27].

The formalin test assesses nociception as well as inflammation. Injection of formalin induces a biphasic response; the early first phase is neurogenic, and results from direct stimulation of nociceptors. This leads to the activation of sensory C-fibers through the transient receptor potential A1 receptors [28] in the paw, and the consequent release of substance P and bradykinin [29]. The late phase is inflammatory, and is due to the release of histamine, serotonin, bradykinin, prostaglandins, sympathomimetic amines, tumor necrosis factor-alpha and interleukins [30,31]. Central sensitization is partly responsible for the prolonged second phase of this test [32].

MSG administered in a dose of 300 mg/kg determined a significant increase in the mean reaction time vs. the control group for phase 2 of the formalin test. More importantly, a similar pattern of nociceptive response was seen during the normally quiet intermediate phase, as in the late phase of the formalin test. This may suggest MSG treatment shifts the tonic phase of formalin nociception to an earlier time point, possibly by enhancing the processes involved in mediating the sensitization in the spinal cord. Data from the literature support our findings regarding the correlation between the administration of MSG and the results of the formalin test. The enhancement of hyperalgesia in rats treated with L-glutamate was reversed by pretreatment with L-NAME. L-glutamate enhances hyperalgesia and persistent nociception following formalin-induced tissue injury, which seems to be mediated by intracellular messengers, including nitric oxide. Intrathecal pretreatment with inhibitors of nitric oxide synthase reduced formalin injury-induced nociceptive behaviors. L-NAME affected the tonic, but not the acute, phase of the formalin response. Conversely, formalin-induced nociceptive responses were enhanced by stimulators of nitric oxide such as sodium nitroprusside [33].

The increase in response during the inflammatory phase could be explained by a NO-induced rise in peripheral concentrations of prostaglandin E2 and prostacyclin, a phenomenon reported by several authors [13,16]. This increase was completely impeded by the NOS inhibitors. In vitro assays support the hypothesis that NO activates cyclooxygenases [34]. These results indicate that NO can also induce peripheral hyperalgesia by regulation of the expression and/or activity of cyclooxygenases, resulting in an increase of prostaglandins release.

The implications of MSG consumption could go further than hyperalgesia, since glutamate induces astrocyte mitochondrial apoptosis. Glutamate increased the expression of representative apoptotic markers, including cleaved caspase-8, cleaved caspase-9, and cleaved caspase-3, as well as level key markers in endoplasmic reticulum stress, in primary cultured spinal cord astrocytes [35]. This opens the way for further investigations: Does administration of MSG impacts spinal cord astrocytes? And what would the consequence be, taking into account the multiple roles of these cells in central nervous system CNS, and given that their apoptosis subsequently leads to CNS injury?

Our findings raise some questions regarding the safety of long-term MSG consumption, and represent a good starting point for any clinical tests focused on examining the impact of MSG nutritional intake on hyperalgesia.

One of these questions concerns the possible interactions between MSG and some analgesics; opioids, non-steroidal anti-inflammatory drugs, and natural products have peripheral and central antinociceptive effect mediated via L-arginine/NO-cGMP pathway [36,37]. Ventura-Martinez et al. showed that acute or chronic administration of L-arginine to mice decreases morphine analgesia. The inhibitory effect of L-arginine on morphine-analgesia and entry into the CNS is blocked by the NOS inhibitor L-NNA [38].

Another issue regards the effect of MSG consumption on pain perception in healthy humans, as well as in those suffering from maladies involving chronic pain. Already, this food additive is classified as a causative substance of headache in the International Classification of Headache Disorders, 3rd edition (ICHD-III beta), and has been found to increase the frequency of fibromyalgia symptoms [7]. Further studies need to be made in order to evaluate the impact of MSG consumption on pain associated with injuries, nerve lesions and degenerative diseases such as osteoarthritis.

Acknowledgments: The authors acknowledge the financial support offered by Romanian National Authority for Scientific Research UEFISCDI through grant PN-II-RU-TE-2014-4-1670, No. 342/2015. The costs to publish in open access were supported by the aforementioned grant.

Author Contributions: A.Z. literature research, performed the pharmacological assays, article preparation; A.N.C. experimental design of pharmacological tests; G.M.N. statistical analysis, literature research, article preparation; B.S.V. performed the biological assays; D.G. development of biochemical assays.

Conflicts of Interest: The authors declare no conflict of interest. The founding sponsors had no role in the design of the study; in the collection, analyses, or interpretation of data; in the writing of the manuscript, and in the decision to publish the results.

References

1. Kwok, R.H.M. Chinese-Restaurant Syndrome. *N. Engl. J. Med.* **1968**, *278*, 796. [PubMed]
2. Evaluation of Food Additives. Specifications for the identity and purity of food additives and their toxocological evaluation: Some extraction solvents and certain other substances; and a review of the technological efficacy of some antimicrobial agents. *World Health Organ. Tech. Rep. Ser.* **1971**, *462*, 1–36.
3. Joint FAO/WHO Expert Committee on Food Additives; World Health Organization; Food and Agriculture Organization of the United Nations. Toxicological evaluation of certain food additives with a review of general principles and of specifications. Seventeenth report of the joint FAO-WHO Expert Committee on Food Additives. *World Health Organ. Tech. Rep. Ser.* **1974**, *539*, 1–40.
4. Walker, R.; Lupien, J.R. The safety evaluation of monosodium glutamate. *J. Nutr.* **2000**, *130*, 1049S–1052S. [PubMed]

5.   Beyreuther, K.; Biesalski, H.K.; Fernstrom, J.D.; Grimm, P.; Hammes, W.P.; Heinemann, U.; Kempski, O.; Stehle, P.; Steinhart, H.; Walker, R. Consensus meeting: Monosodium glutamate—An update. *Eur. J. Clin. Nutr.* **2006**, *61*, 304–313. [CrossRef] [PubMed]

6.   Shimada, A.; Baad-Hansen, L.; Castrillon, E.; Ghafouri, B.; Stensson, N.; Gerdle, B.; Ernberg, M.; Cairns, B.; Svensson, P.; Svensson Odont, P. Differential effects of repetitive oral administration of monosodium glutamate on interstitial glutamate concentration and muscle pain sensitivity. *Nutrition* **2015**, *31*, 315–323. [CrossRef] [PubMed]

7.   Holton, K.F.; Taren, D.L.; Thomson, C.A.; Bennett, R.M.; Jones, K.D. The effect of dietary glutamate on fibromyalgia and irritable bowel symptoms. *Clin. Exp. Rheumatol.* **2012**, *30*, 10–17. [PubMed]

8.   Hoffman, E.M.; Zhang, Z.; Schechter, R.; Miller, K.E. Glutaminase increases in rat dorsal root ganglion neurons after unilateral adjuvant-induced hind paw inflammation. *Biomolecules* **2016**, *6*, 10. [CrossRef] [PubMed]

9.   Szekely, J.I.; Torok, K.; Mate, G. The Role of Ionotropic Glutamate Receptors in Nociception with Special Regard to the AMPA Binding Sites. *Curr. Pharm. Des.* **2002**, *8*, 887–912. [CrossRef] [PubMed]

10. Larsson, M. Ionotropic Glutamate Receptors in Spinal Nociceptive Processing. *Mol. Neurobiol.* **2009**, *40*, 260–288. [CrossRef] [PubMed]

11. Neugebauer, V. Metabotropic glutamate receptors–important modulators of nociception and pain behavior. *Pain* **2002**, *98*, 1–8. [CrossRef]

12. Chiechio, S. Chapter Three-Modulation of Chronic Pain by Metabotropic Glutamate Receptors. *Adv. Pharm.* **2016**, *75*, 63–89.

13. Chen, Z.; Muscoli, C.; Doyle, T.; Bryant, L.; Cuzzocrea, S.; Mollace, V.; Mastroianni, R.; Masini, E.; Salvemini, D. NMDA receptor activation and nitroxidative regulation of the glutamatergic pathway during nociceptive processing. *Pain* **2010**, *149*, 100–106. [CrossRef] [PubMed]

14. Gangadharan, V.; Wang, R.; Ulzhöfer, B.; Luo, C.; Bardoni, R.; Bali, K.K.; Agarwal, N.; Tegeder, I.; Hildebrandt, U.; Nagy, G.G.; et al. Peripheral calcium-permeable AMPA receptors regulate chronic inflammatory pain in mice. *J. Clin. Investig.* **2011**, *121*, 1608–1623. [CrossRef] [PubMed]

15. Luo, Z.D.; Cizkova, D. The role of nitric oxide in nociception. *Curr. Rev. Pain* **2000**, *4*, 459–466. [CrossRef] [PubMed]

16. Toriyabe, M.; Omote, K.; Kawamata, T.; Namiki, A. Contribution of Interaction between Nitric Oxide and Cyclooxygenases to the Production of Prostaglandins in Carrageenan-induced Inflammation. *Anesthesiology* **2004**, *101*, 983–990. [CrossRef] [PubMed]

17. Damasceno, F.; Skinner, G.O.; Araújo, P.C.; Ferraz, M.M.D.; Tenório, F.; de Almeida, O.M.M.S. Nitric oxide modulates the hyperalgesic response to mechanical noxious stimuli in sleep-deprived rats. *BMC Neurosci.* **2013**, *14*, 92. [CrossRef] [PubMed]

18. Kuboyama, K.; Tsuda, M.; Tsutsui, M.; Toyohara, Y.; Tozaki-Saitoh, H.; Shimokawa, H.; Yanagihara, N.; Inoue, K. Reduced spinal microglial activation and neuropathic pain after nerve injury in mice lacking all three nitric oxide synthases. *Mol. Pain* **2011**, *7*, 50. [CrossRef] [PubMed]

19. Yoon, Y.W.; Sung, B.; Chung, J.M. Nitric oxide mediates behavioral signs of neuropathic pain in an experimental rat model. *Neuroreport* **1998**, *9*, 367–372. [CrossRef] [PubMed]

20. Chacur, M.; Matos, R.J.B.; Alves, A.S.; Rodrigues, A.C.; Gutierrez, V.; Cury, Y.; Britto, L.R.G. Participation of neuronal nitric oxide synthase in experimental neuropathic pain induced by sciatic nerve transection. *Brazilian J. Med. Biol. Res.* **2010**, *43*, 367–376. [CrossRef] [PubMed]

21. Chen, Y.; Boettger, M.K.; Reif, A.; Schmitt, A.; Üçeyler, N.; Sommer, C. Nitric oxide synthase modulates CFA-induced thermal hyperalgesia through cytokine regulation in mice. *Mol. Pain* **2010**, *6*, 13. [CrossRef] [PubMed]

22. Buzescu, A.; Negres, S.; Călin, O.; Chirită, C. Experimental demonstration of hyperalgesia induced by repeated ingestion of dietary monosodium glutamate. *Farmacia* **2013**, *61*, 1009–1017.

23. Tsikas, D. Analysis of nitrite and nitrate in biological fluids by assays based on the Griess reaction: Appraisal of the Griess reaction in the L-arginine/nitric oxide area of research. *J. Chromatogr. B* **2007**, *851*, 51–70. [CrossRef] [PubMed]

24. Krohn, R.I. The Colorimetric Detection and Quantitation of Total Protein. In *Current Protocols in Cell Biology*; John Wiley & Sons, Inc.: Hoboken, NJ, USA, 2001.

25. Gunn, A.; Bobeck, E.N.; Weber, C.; Morgan, M.M. The influence of non-nociceptive factors on hot-plate latency in rats. *J. Pain* **2011**, *12*, 222–227. [CrossRef] [PubMed]

26. De Sousa, D.P. Analgesic-like activity of essential oils constituents. *Molecules* **2011**, *16*, 2233–2252. [CrossRef] [PubMed]

27. Cury, Y.; Picolo, G.; Gutierrez, V.P.; Ferreira, S.H. Pain and analgesia: The dual effect of nitric oxide in the nociceptive system. *Nitric Oxide* **2011**, *25*, 243–254. [CrossRef] [PubMed]

28. McNamara, C.R.; Mandel-Brehm, J.; Bautista, D.M.; Siemens, J.; Deranian, K.L.; Zhao, M.; Hayward, N.J.; Chong, J.A.; Julius, D.; Moran, M.M.; et al. TRPA1 mediates formalin-induced pain. *Proc. Natl. Acad. Sci. USA* **2007**, *104*, 13525–13530. [CrossRef] [PubMed]

29. Parada, C.A.; Tambeli, C.H.; Cunha, F.Q.; Ferreira, S.H. The major role of peripheral release of histamine and 5-hydroxytryptamine in formalin-induced nociception. *Neuroscience* **2001**, *102*, 937–944. [CrossRef]

30. Milano, J.; Oliveira, S.M.; Rossato, M.F.; Sauzem, P.D.; Machado, P.; Beck, P.; Zanatta, N.; Martins, M.A.P.; Mello, C.F.; Rubin, M.A.; et al. Antinociceptive effect of novel trihalomethyl-substituted pyrazoline methyl esters in formalin and hot-plate tests in mice. *Eur. J. Pharmacol.* **2008**, *581*, 86–96. [CrossRef] [PubMed]

31. Zeashan, H.; Amresh, G.; Rao, C.V.; Singh, S. Antinociceptive activity of Amaranthus spinosus in experimental animals. *J. Ethnopharmacol.* **2009**, *122*, 492–496. [CrossRef] [PubMed]

32. Coderre, T.J.; Melzack, R. The contribution of excitatory amino acids to central sensitization and persistent nociception after formalin-induced tissue injury. *J. Neurosci.* **1992**, *12*, 3665–3670. [PubMed]

33. Coderre, T.J.; Yashpal, K. Intracellular Messengers Contributing to Persistent Nociception and Hyperalgesia Induced by L-Glutamate and Substance P in the Rat Formalin Pain Model. *Eur. J. Neurosci.* **1994**, *6*, 1328–1334. [CrossRef] [PubMed]

34. Little, J.W.; Doyle, T.; Salvemini, D. Reactive nitroxidative species and nociceptive processing: Determining the roles for nitric oxide, superoxide, and peroxynitrite in pain. *Amino Acids* **2012**, *42*, 75–94. [CrossRef] [PubMed]

35. Zhang, C.; Wang, C.; Ren, J.; Guo, X.; Yun, K. Morphine Protects Spinal Cord Astrocytes from Glutamate-Induced Apoptosis via Reducing Endoplasmic Reticulum Stress. *Int. J. Mol. Sci.* **2016**, *17*, 1523. [CrossRef] [PubMed]

36. Ventura-Martínez, R.; Déciga-Campos, M.; Díaz-Reval, M.I.; González-Trujano, M.E.; López-Muñoz, F.J. Peripheral involvement of the nitric oxide-cGMP pathway in the indomethacin-induced antinociception in rat. *Eur. J. Pharmacol.* **2004**, *503*, 43–48. [CrossRef] [PubMed]

37. Déciga-Campos, M.; López-Muñoz, F.J. Participation of the L-arginine-nitric oxide-cyclic GMP-ATP-sensitive K$^+$ channel cascade in the antinociceptive effect of rofecoxib. *Eur. J. Pharmacol.* **2004**, *484*, 193–199. [CrossRef] [PubMed]

38. Hishikawa, K.; Nakaki, T.; Tsuda, M.; Esumi, H.; Ohshima, H.; Suzuki, H.; Saruta, T.; Kato, R. Effect of systemic L-arginine administration on hemodynamics and nitric oxide release in man. *Jpn. Heart J.* **1992**, *33*, 41–48. [CrossRef] [PubMed]

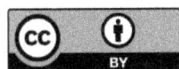

© 2017 by the authors. Licensee MDPI, Basel, Switzerland. This article is an open access article distributed under the terms and conditions of the Creative Commons Attribution (CC BY) license (http://creativecommons.org/licenses/by/4.0/).

nutrients

MDPI

Article

Dietary Sialyllactose Does Not Influence Measures of Recognition Memory or Diurnal Activity in the Young Pig

Stephen A. Fleming [1,2], Maciej Chichlowski [3], Brian M. Berg [3,4], Sharon M. Donovan [4,5] and Ryan N. Dilger [1,2,4,*]

[1] Piglet Nutrition and Cognition Laboratory, Department of Animal Sciences, University of Illinois, Urbana, IL 61801, USA; sflemin2@illinois.edu

[2] Department of Animal Sciences, University of Illinois, Urbana, IL 61801, USA

[3] Mead Johnson Pediatric Nutrition Institute, Evansville, IL 61142, USA; maciej.chichlowski@rb.com (M.C.); dr.brianberg@gmail.com (B.M.B.)

[4] Division of Nutritional Sciences, University of Illinois, Urbana, IL 61801, USA; sdonovan@illinois.edu

[5] Department of Food Science and Human Nutrition, University of Illinois Urbana-Champaign, Urbana, IL 61801, USA

* Correspondence: rdilger2@illinois.edu; Tel.: +1-(217)-333-2006

Received: 29 January 2018; Accepted: 21 March 2018; Published: 23 March 2018

Abstract: Sialic acid (SA) is an integral component of gangliosides and signaling molecules in the brain and its dietary intake may support cognitive development. We previously reported that feeding sialyllactose, a milk oligosaccharide that contains SA, alters SA content and diffusivity in the pig brain. The present research sought to expand upon such results and describe the effects of feeding sialyllactose on recognition memory and sleep/wake activity using a translational pig model. Pigs were provided ad libitum access to a customized milk replacer containing 0 g/L or 380 g/L of sialyllactose from postnatal day (PND) 2–22. Beginning on PND 15, pigs were fitted with accelerometers to track home-cage activity and testing on the novel object recognition task began at PND 17. There were no significant effects of diet on average daily body weight gain, average daily milk intake, or the gain-to-feed ratio during the study (all $p \geq 0.11$). Pigs on both diets were able to display recognition memory on the novel object recognition task ($p < 0.01$), but performance and exploratory behavior did not differ between groups (all $p \geq 0.11$). Total activity and percent time spent sleeping were equivalent between groups during both day and night cycles (all $p \geq 0.56$). Dietary sialyllactose did not alter growth performance of young pigs, and there was no evidence that providing SA via sialyllactose benefits the development of recognition memory or gross sleep-related behaviors.

Keywords: pig; nutrition; brain; development; sialyllactose; sialic acid; oligosaccharide; cognition

1. Introduction

Human milk has been shown to have numerous benefits in comparison to infant formula in stimulating the growth and development of gastrointestinal and immune systems [1]. A recent meta-analysis suggests that breastfeeding promotes cognitive development [2], but the mechanisms and strength of the relationship are unclear [3]. There is mounting evidence that components of human milk such as DHA [4], choline [5], and gangliosides [6] support brain development, and emerging research suggests milk oligosaccharides (ranging from 3–32 monosaccharide units in length [7]) may contribute to brain development as well [8]. Some milk oligosaccharides may act as prebiotics [8], and we recently demonstrated that pigs fed a combination of prebiotics demonstrated increased exploratory behavior and improved recognition memory [9]. Milk oligosaccharides are a heterogeneous group of oligosaccharides with diverse functions largely related to immunity and gut physiology [8]. The composition of human milk oligosaccharides is 10–20% sialylated [8]. As sialic acid (SA) is present at relatively high concentrations in the brain as a part of gangliosides and signaling molecules that regulate neurodevelopment [6], the impact of sialylated oligosaccharides such as sialyllactose (SL) is of interest as they may support brain development.

Supplementation with SA-containing ingredients, including complex milk lipids [10], gangliosides [11], casein glycomacropeptide (cGMP) [12], lactoferrin [13], and SL [14], has been shown to improve cognition or alter stress-related behaviors. In a young adult mouse model investigating possible anxiolytic effects of SL, both 3′ and 6′ isomers reduced anxiety-related measures and restored performance to control levels when mice were introduced to a social stressor. Furthermore, SL attenuated stress-related sleep disruptions in adult rats [15] and tended to increase performance on spatially-based behavioral tasks [16]. A recent study demonstrated that pigs fed SL-supplemented formula for 21 days had greater total SA concentrations in the corpus callosum when fed milk containing 2 g/L of either 3′- or 6′-SL compared with pigs provided formula containing no SL or 4 g SL/L milk [17]. Similarly, a previous study from our lab showed that of a range of doses of SL, ranging from 55–779 mg SL/L of formula, a moderate dosage of 429 mg SL/L increased free-to-bound hippocampal SA, reduced bound SA in the prefrontal cortex, and increased mean, axial, and radial diffusivity in the corpus callosum [18]. Taken together with the findings of Jacobi and colleagues [17], these results show that feeding SL results in dose-dependent, structural, and region-specific increases in brain SA, but it remains to be shown whether this has functional consequences for behavior. Accordingly, our hypothesis in the present study was that supplementation with a moderate dosage of 380 mg SL/L would improve the performance of pigs on the novel object recognition task and influence measures of sleep/wake activity. We chose to supplement the diet at 380 mg SL/L, which is within the concentration range found in mature human milk [19].

2. Materials and Methods

2.1. Animals and Housing

All animal care and experimental procedures were in accordance with the National Research Council Guide for the Care and Use of Laboratory Animals and approved by the University of Illinois at Urbana-Champaign Institutional Animal Care and Use Committee. Approval for this research project was verified on 3 March 2015 and is identified as IACUC 15034 at the University of Illinois Urbana-Champaign. Beginning on postnatal day (PND) 2, naturally-farrowed, intact male pigs ($n = 36$) were artificially-reared through PND 22. The trial was completed in one replicate with 18 pigs per diet, selected from 9 L to control for genetics (same sire and related dams between litters) and initial bodyweight. All pigs were provided a single subcutaneous 5 mL dose of *Clostridium perfringens* antitoxin C and D (Colorado Serum Company, Denver, CO, USA) on PND 2. If health status appeared compromised (i.e., diarrhea, lethargy, elevated body temperature), an additional 5 mL dose of *C. perfringens* antitoxin C and D was administered orally until symptoms resolved; a total of seven pigs were given additional doses of antitoxin. Housing, temperature, and lighting were conducted as described previously [18]. Two pigs were euthanized prior to the conclusion of the study due to insufficient weight gain and failure-to-thrive ($n = 1$/diet). Data from the remaining 34 pigs ($n = 17$/diet) were used for subsequent analyses and are presented herein.

2.2. Dietary Groups

All diets were produced by Mead Johnson Nutrition (Evansville, IN, USA) using a proprietary blend of nutrients formulated to meet the nutritional needs of growing pigs. Pigs were provided one of two custom diets from PND 2–22. The control diet (Control) included docosahexaenoic acid (DHA, 87 mg/100 g milk replacer powder; DSM, Heerlen, The Netherlands), arachidonic acid (ARA, 174 mg/100 g milk replacer powder; DSM, Heerlen, The Netherlands), galactooligosaccharide (GOS,

1.0 g/100 g milk replacer powder; FrieslandCampina, Zwolle, The Netherlands), and polydextrose (PDX, 1.0 g/100 g milk replacer powder; Danisco, Terre Haute, IN, USA). The experimental diet (Sialyllactose) was formulated using the Control diet as the base and supplemented with bovine-derived modified whey enriched with SL (SAL-10; Arla Foods Ingredients, Aarhus, Denmark) to provide a final SL concentration of 190 mg SL/100 g milk replacer powder.

Milk replacer powder was reconstituted fresh each day at 200 g of dry powder per 800 g of water. At this reconstitution rate, all diets provided equal concentrations of DHA (174 mg/L), ARA (348 mg/L), and PDX/GOS (each at 2 g/L). The reconstituted milk replacers were formulated to contain 0 mg SL/L (Control) or 380 mg SL/L (Sialyllactose). Pigs were fed ad libitum using an automated milk replacer delivery system that dispensed milk from 10:00 to 06:00 the next day. Leftover milk from the previous day and individual pig bodyweights were recorded daily. The remaining volume of milk was subtracted from the initial volume provided to quantify milk disappearance following the 20-h feeding period, which will henceforth be referred to as milk intake. Milk intake from PND 21 was omitted from analyses as pigs were fasted overnight prior to the end of study on PND 22. An electrolyte solution (Swine Bluelite, Tech Mix, Stewart, MN, USA) was provided to all pigs from PND 2–5 to help maintain electrolyte balance and avoid dehydration.

2.3. Behavioral Testing

2.3.1. Novel Object Recognition

The novel object recognition (NOR) task was used to assess object recognition memory. Testing consisted of a habituation phase, a sample phase, and a test phase. During the habituation phase, each pig was placed in an empty testing arena for 10 min each day for two days leading up to the sample phase. In the sample phase, the pig was placed in the arena containing two identical objects and given 5 min for exploration. After a delay of 48 h, the pig was returned to the arena for the test phase. During the test phase, the pig was placed in the arena containing one object from the sample phase as well as a novel object and allowed to explore for 5 min. Between trials, objects were removed, immersed in hot water with detergent and rubbed with a towel to mitigate odor, and the arena was sprayed with water to remove urine and feces. Objects chosen had a range of characteristics (i.e., color, texture, shape, and size); however, the novel and sample objects only differed in shape and size. Only objects previously shown to elicit a null preference were used for testing. Habituation trials began at PND 17 and testing on the NOR task began at PND 19. The amount of time exploring objects and distance moved was measured using a combination of automated procedures using Ethovision (Ethovision XT 11[®], Noldus Information Technology, Wageningen, The Netherlands) and manual tracking (for a review of each measure assessed, see Fleming and Dilger [20]). The recognition index, the proportion of time spent with the novel object compared to total exploration of both objects, was used to measure recognition memory. A recognition index significantly above 0.50 demonstrates a novelty preference and, thus, recognition memory. Trials were removed from analyses if experimental/technical errors existed or pigs explored either object for less than 2 s during the sample or test trial. If pigs did not explore either object for greater than 2 s during the sample trial, they were also removed from analysis during the test trial regardless of performance. Two and five pigs provided the Control and SL diets, respectively, did not meet the above criteria and were removed from the final analysis (final $n = 15$, Control; $n = 12$, Sialyllactose).

2.3.2. Activity Analysis

Accelerometers (Actiwatch 2, Philips Respironics, Bend, OR, USA) were secured to collars and fastened around each pig's neck between PND 15 and 22 ($n = 12$ per diet) and were set to sample movement every 15 s. Only periods where full day and night cycles were recorded were used for analysis (PND 15 and 22 were omitted as collars were only on for part of the day, for a remaining total of six full cycles between PND 16 and 21). When pigs were found without collars, the collar was re-applied and the time was noted. After study completion, home-cage video was used to verify that periods of complete inactivity were due to the loss of the collar, and these times were also removed from analysis. For the analysis of sleep/wake outcomes, specialized software (Actiware 6.0.7, Philips Respironics, Murrysville, PA, USA) was used to calculate a unique wake threshold value (used to determine if the pig was asleep or awake based on movement during 2-min periods before and after a single 15-s epoch) for each pig and quantify the total activity count and percent time asleep. Data were collected for six consecutive days and sleep outcomes were assessed as averages across that period.

A preliminary analysis was conducted to assess the validity of sleep scores in pigs from actigraphy data. Approximately one hour of activity data collected from six pigs was scored by actigraphy software as compared to the manual scoring of recorded video. Video was split into 15-s epochs, for a total of 247 epochs, and manually analyzed. If a pig was visually-assessed as asleep for more than 50% of a single 15-s epoch, that epoch was classified as a "sleep" epoch. Epochs were chosen by selecting for periods of apparent transition between sleep and wakefulness as these are the most difficult to classify and appeared to be most variable between manual and automatic scoring methods.

2.4. Statistical Analysis

All data generated as part of this study were subjected to an analysis of variance (ANOVA) using the MIXED procedure of SAS Enterprise Guide 5.1 (SAS Institute Inc., Cary, NC, USA). Depending on the outcome, one of two statistical models was used: (1) data collected at a single time-point (e.g., average body weight gain over the entire study, performance in the NOR test trial) were analyzed by one-way ANOVA; and (2) data collected from the same animal on more than one occasion (e.g., diurnal activity) were analyzed using two-way repeated-measures ANOVA. Litter was included as a random effect in both statistical models. For NOR testing, a one-tailed t-test was conducted to assess if recognition index was greater than 0.5 (i.e., random chance). In all instances statistical significance was considered at $p < 0.05$.

3. Results

3.1. Diet Composition

Analytical assessment conducted after study completion showed levels of SL in the experimental diets were close to formulated levels (374 mg SL/L vs. 380 mg SL/L in the Sialyllactose diet). However, the Control diet contained 58 mg SL/L due to endogenous SL in the bovine milk ingredients. Energy, macronutrient, and micronutrient composition were comparable between Control and Sialyllactose diets (see Table 1 for analyzed nutrient composition).

Table 1. Analyzed nutrient composition of experimental diets.

Nutrient per Liter	Control	Sialyllactose
Sialyllactose, mg	58	374
Energy and macronutrients		
Total calories, kcal	1049	1020
Carbohydrate, g	57	58
Fat, g	64	60
Protein, g	61	62
Minerals		
Calcium, mg	2233	2178
Chlorine, mg	1141	1158
Copper, µg	1640	1505
Iodine, µg	274	271
Iron, mg	19	19
Magnesium, mg	227	241

Table 1. *Cont.*

Nutrient per Liter	Control	Sialyllactose
Manganese, µg	2305	2159
Phosphorus, mg	1621	1673
Potassium, mg	2255	2349
Selenium, µg	65	68
Sodium, mg	1708	1708
Zinc, mg	17	17
Vitamins and other nutrients		
Vitamin A, IU	4572	4112
Vitamin D_3, IU	761	795
Vitamin E, IU	30	31
Vitamin K, µg	321	362
Thiamin, µg	1322	1588
Riboflavin, µg	2608	2780
Niacin, µg	13,366	11,132
Vitamin B_6, µg	1210	1414
Folic acid, µg	211	237
Vitamin B_{12}, µg	6	7
Pantothenic acid, µg	9216	8170
Biotin, µg	74	74
Choline, mg	352	394
Polydextrose, g	1.8	1.9
Galactooligosaccharide, g	2.1	1.7
Arachidonic acid, mg	318	288
Docosahexaenoic acid, mg	155	141

3.2. Growth Performance and Health Status

No differences were observed for average daily body weight gain, average daily milk intake, or the feed efficiency ratio (i.e., gain-to-milk intake) between diets across the duration of the study (all $p \geq 0.11$, Table 2, Figure 1). Additionally, daily health checks revealed low incidence of loose stool in pigs and no differences in pig health status or compliance to consume experimental dietary treatments. Thus, all pigs remained healthy throughout the study duration and both dietary treatments were equally well tolerated by pigs as evident in the observed trajectory of body weight gain.

Table 2. Effects of dietary sialyllactose supplementation on the growth performance of pigs over the duration of the feeding study [1].

| | Diet [2] | | Pooled | |
Measure [3]	Control	Sialyllactose	SEM	*p*-Value [4]
ADG, g/day	311	306	14	0.69
ADMI, g milk/day	1220	1347	62	0.11
ADMI, g solids/day	244	269	12	0.11
G:F, g BW:kg milk	255	234	11	0.16

[1] Abbreviations: SEM, standard error of the mean; BW, body weight; kg, kilogram; ADG, average daily body weight gain; ADMI, average daily milk intake; G:F, gain-to-feed ratio (i.e., feed efficiency); [2] $n = 17$ per diet; [3] Calculations reflect a milk reconstitution rate of 20% solids; [4] *p*-values derived from mixed model ANOVA.

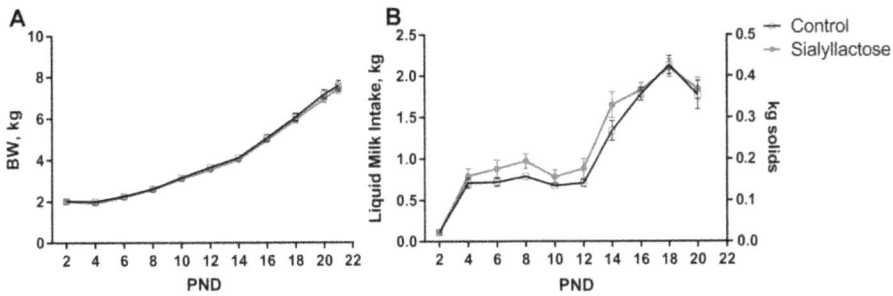

Figure 1. Body weight (BW) (**A**) and liquid milk intake (**B**) during the trial. No differences in average daily body weight gain, average daily milk intake, or the feed efficiency ratio (i.e., body weight gain:feed intake ratio) were observed between groups ($p \geq 0.11$). Data for milk intake on postnatal day (PND) 22 are not shown as piglets were fasted overnight prior to the end of study.

3.3. Novel Object Recognition

Regardless of dietary treatment, all pigs were able to display recognition memory in the NOR test trial ($p < 0.01$, Table 3). However, there were no differences between dietary treatment groups for measures of exploratory behavior, most notably time spent investigating objects, number of object visits, and mean time spent per object visit (all $p \geq 0.11$, Table 4). Although some pigs were removed due to non-compliance, ultimately our study was powered to capture an effect size of 0.89 with a power of 0.80 when evaluating differences in the NOR recognition index.

Table 3. Ability of pigs to display a recognition index score above 0.50 as a measure of recognition memory in the NOR test trial [1].

Diet	n	Mean	SEM	p-Value [2]
Control	15	0.65	0.046	<0.01
Sialyllactose	12	0.66	0.047	<0.01

[1] Abbreviations: NOR, novel object recognition; SEM, standard error of the mean; [2] p-Value derived from one-tailed *t*-test for a recognition index above 0.50.

Table 4. Effect of dietary sialyllactose supplementation on exploratory behavior during the test trial of the NOR task [1].

				Diet			
			Control		Sialyllactose	Pooled	
Measure		n	Mean	n	Mean	SEM	p-Value [2]
Recognition index		15	0.66	12	0.65	0.05	0.94
Novel object visit time, s		15	56.63	12	42.05	7.77	0.18
Number of novel object visits		15	8.33	12	6.78	1.07	0.25
Mean novel object visit time, s		15	6.19	11	6.41	1.12	0.88
Latency to first novel object visit, s		15	25.46	12	25.32	9.31	0.99
Habituation towards the novel object, s/min		15	−1.60	12	−0.69	1.25	0.59
Sample object visit time, s		14	28.27	12	22.45	6.45	0.50
Number of sample object visits		15	4.77	12	4.62	0.56	0.84
Mean sample object visit time, s		15	6.18	12	5.51	1.34	0.71
Latency to first sample object visit, s		14	24.08	12	14.25	7.15	0.31
Habituation towards the sample object, s/min		14	−2.68	12	−1.78	0.73	0.35
Total object visit time, s		15	82.52	12	70.35	13.51	0.47
Mean object visit time, s		15	7.10	12	6.11	1.22	0.55

Table 4. *Cont.*

Measure	Control		Sialyllactose		Pooled	
	n	Mean	*n*	Mean	SEM	*p*-Value [2]
Number of object visits	15	13.13	12	11.42	1.34	0.31
Latency to first object visit, s	15	9.48	12	13.50	4.97	0.55
Habituation towards both objects, s/min	15	−4.32	12	−1.76	1.39	0.19
Total distance moved, m	15	2.43	11	2.11	0.19	0.11
Time spent in the center of the arena, %	15	58.76	12	56.73	6.95	0.80

[1] Abbreviations: NOR, novel object recognition; SEM, standard error of the mean; [2] *p*-Values derived from mixed model ANOVA.

3.4. Activity Analysis

Validation of the automated scoring method (i.e., computer-assisted analysis of actigraphy data) against the manual scoring of home-cage video was performed. A chi-square test for equality of two proportions showed that automated and manual scoring methods were not different ($p = 0.065$), with the automated scoring being only 7% more likely to score an epoch as "sleep" and less likely to score an epoch as "awake". Therefore, with the validation of the automated actigraphy data scoring method complete, all sleep/wake activity reported herein was generated using the automated software-based method. In general, there was no significant main effect of diet or interaction effect of diet by cycle for total activity or percent time asleep (all $p \geq 0.56$, Table 5). While intuitive, total activity counts and time asleep were both influenced by cycle (i.e., day vs. night; both $p < 0.01$).

Table 5. Effect of dietary sialyllactose supplementation on diurnal activity of pigs [1].

Measure	Control				Sialyllactose				Pooled	*p*-Value [3]		
	Day		Night		Day		Night					
	n	Mean	*n*	Mean	*n*	Mean	*n*	Mean	SEM	Diet	Cycle	Interaction
Total activity count	65	1.6×10^5	70	6.9×10^4	67	1.7×10^5	72	6.9×10^4	7.0×10^3	0.64	<0.01	0.56
Time asleep, %	65	67.47	70	84.90	71	67.43	72	85.63	0.97	0.61	<0.01	0.58

[1] Abbreviations: SEM, standard error of the mean; %, percent; [2] Data from 12 pigs per diet over a six-day period; [3] *p*-Value derived from repeated measures mixed model ANOVA.

4. Discussion

Siallylactose is one of several sources of SA, and comparisons of mature human and porcine milk demonstrate that the SA content of human milk is much greater than that of porcine milk. Mature human milk provides approximately 500 mg SA/L milk [21], porcine milk contains approximately 10 mg SA/L milk [22], and infant formula falls between 65–290 mg SA/L milk [23] (for a thorough review of SA content of milk and other food products, see Röhrig et al. [24]). In this study, a dose of 380 mg SL/L was tested as a previous study reported that this dose was most effective at eliciting changes in SA content and diffusivity in the brain [18]. This dose is well below the SL dose that was shown by Jacobi et al. [17] to enrich corpus callosum and hippocampal SA content [17], but is within the range found in mature human milk [19]. Here, the impact of dietary SL on growth, recognition memory, exploratory behavior, and diurnal activity was investigated, but no impact of diet was observed for any measure.

Pigs fed an SL-supplemented diet did not display altered sleep behavior, whereas a past report demonstrated that SL attenuated disruptions to sleep architecture after exposure to an acute inescapable stress [15]. An important distinction from past research is that diurnal activity was measured in a minimally stressful environment, whereas SL may provide a neuroprotective effect that is only observed in the context of a more extreme stressor. Additionally, Chichlowski et al. [15] used electroencephalography (EEG), allowing the experimenters to more accurately quantify the timing, stage, and quality of sleep. Although both treatment groups in our study had similar activity during the day and night, differences in the quality of sleep may have been observed if assessments were made using EEG.

While different doses and/or longer duration of SL administration may have produced a cognitive benefit, it is possible that supplemental SA (via SL) was not required in the behavioral paradigm under which the pigs were assessed. Active learning increases the expression of mRNA for the enzyme critical for regulating SA biosynthesis (UDP-N-acetylglucoasamine-2-epimerase/N-acetylmannosamine kinase, GNE) by 2- to 3-fold in the hippocampus and liver of pigs [25]. As the NOR task makes use of spontaneous behavior rather than operant conditioning the cognitive load required to learn a rule was not present, and there may not have been a physiological demand for increased SA utilization in the brain. Our data show that dietary SL supplementation did not provide a cognitive benefit as assessed by NOR, which conflicts with previous work that showed young pigs exhibit cognitive benefits from dietary SA supplementation when using behavioral tasks dependent on operant conditioning [12,13]. Moreover, these results may reflect the presence of prebiotics in both the control and experimental diet. We previously reported that pigs fed milk replacers containing the prebiotics PDX and GOS demonstrated increased exploratory behavior and improved recognition memory using the same behavioral paradigm (i.e., the NOR task with a delay of 48 h) [9]. Together with evidence that piglets are capable of performing the NOR task at younger ages using shorter delays [20], we believe the difficulty of the task was appropriate. Rather, the potential cognitive benefits from SL may have been masked by the inclusion of PDX and GOS in each diet.

To our knowledge, few studies have evaluated the ability of dietary SL to affect behavior and cognition. Tarr and colleagues [14] found that dietary SL attenuated stressor induced anxiety-like behaviors in rats and preliminary data suggests that SL may prevent stress-induced alterations in sleep architecture [15]. However, another report in rats demonstrated that feeding SL only produced a non-significant trend towards improved cognition on spatial tasks [16]. The majority of data suggesting dietary SL may be beneficial for cognitive development come indirectly from studies that investigated other SA-containing ingredients such as gangliosides [10,11,26], cGMP [12], and lactoferrin [13]. Each of these ingredients vary in structure and function, but are common in that they contain SA. Gangliosides are sialylated glycosphingolipids highly concentrated in the brain [6], cGMP is an SA-enriched peptide released during the formation of cheese from the protein kappa-casein [27], and lactoferrin is an iron binding glycoprotein enriched in SA with various functions related to iron metabolism [28].

Gangliosides contribute 75% of conjugated SA in the brain where they play a critical role in functions such as synaptic transmission, plasticity, neurogenesis, synaptogenesis, cell proliferation, and cell differentiation [6]. Exogenous, but not dietary, gangliosides and SA appear to be effective at promoting cognition in adult or aging models [29–33] and deficit (i.e., drug-induced amnesia, cortical lesions, malnourishment) models [34–36]. The impact on young, normal animals is mixed, but ganglioside and SA administration have shown both positive and neutral effects on cognition [31,37]. These studies provided preliminary evidence that exogenous SA improves cognition; however, there is less evidence that dietary gangliosides improve cognition in normative models (i.e., gangliosides are provided at physiological concentrations via the diet to healthy animals during typical development).

Male and female pigs fed formula containing a mix of 0.8% or 2.5% phospholipids and gangliosides displayed fewer errors in a spatial T-maze test compared with controls and had larger brain weights. Furthermore, volumes of several brain regions including the internal capsule, putamen, and thalamus appeared sensitive to supplementation [11]. As has been discussed for SA, the cognitive effects of dietary ganglioside supplementation appear dependent on dosage and behavioral task employed. Rats provided complex milk lipid in doses of 1.0% but not 0.2% exhibited greater behavioral performance in the novel object recognition and Morris water maze, but no improvement in operant conditioning tasks [10]. A subsequent report from the same group demonstrated that even lower doses of 0.05% and 0.01% had no effect on operant learning, and spatial or recognition memory [38]. In a separate study, dietary gangliosides fed to children with cerebral palsy for 3 months elicited improved muscle tension, limb function, language ability, and intelligence [26]. Due to the use of a developmentally-appropriate preclinical model for the human infant, this study provides strong evidence that gangliosides contribute to not only cognition but also motor function and development. Taken together these data suggest that, provided the correct dosage, gangliosides fed alone or as part of a complex milk lipid may have the capacity to promote cognitive development.

Young pigs supplemented with SA via cGMP from PND 3–35 displayed dose-dependent increases in performance in the radial arm maze, with those provided the most cGMP completing the difficult version of the task with the fewest mistakes. All groups fed cGMP had enriched protein-bound, but not ganglioside-bound, SA in the frontal cortex. Additionally, pigs fed the highest amount of cGMP had increased levels of *ST8SIAIV*, a polysialyltransferase important in SA metabolism. After a correlational analysis, it was revealed that sialyltransferase activity in the frontal cortex correlated inversely with number of mistakes on the behavioral task, with pigs exhibiting lower sialyltransferase activity making more mistakes. Despite this correlation, there were no dietary effects on sialyltransferase activity, suggesting sialyltransferase activity may not be involved in the mechanism by which performance was improved. In a later study by the same group, pigs supplemented with lactoferrin from PND 3–38 were found to have increased performance on the radial maze. More pigs in the treatment group were able to complete both easy and difficult versions of the task, with the pigs provided lactoferrin making fewer mistakes on the difficult version [13]. Gene microarray data in hippocampal tissue revealed that pigs fed lactoferrin had upregulated expression of genes in the brain-derived neurotrophic factor (BDNF) neurotrophic signaling pathway, affecting genes related to organization of the cytoplasm, cytoskeleton, growth of neurites, and anxiety [13]. The finding that the provision of dietary lactoferrin influenced the expression of genes related to anxiety suggested that this protein may decrease anxiety, which aligns with the previously discussed results from Tarr et al. [14], wherein mice provided SL demonstrated attenuated anxiety when introduced to a social stressor.

Overall, few studies have evaluated the impact of SL on cognition and behavior. However, there is evidence that SA-containing ingredients positively influence cognitive performance, but making cross-sectional comparisons is confounded by the use of several different SA-enriched ingredients. While containing SA, SL, gangliosides, cGMP, and lactoferrin differ vastly in structure and function, contributing to the variation between study results.

Although our intervention coincided with a significant portion of brain growth in the pig, our investigation may have been limited by the duration of the trial, which may not have allowed sufficient time for SL to confer cognitive benefits. As discussed, the novel object recognition task may not reflect a context wherein supplemental SA is beneficial, and comparisons between spontaneous and operant behavior may elucidate the conditions that lead to increased neural requirements for SA. While clinically translatable, the use of actigraphy instead of EEG did not allow the examination of neural activity during sleep and the quantification of sleep stages, thus our measures were only a gross representation of sleep activity. Lastly, although the goal of this study was to evaluate the efficacy of 380 mg SL/L at supporting cognitive development, we cannot exclude the possibility that a higher supplementation dose or longer supplementation period may have elicited cognitive benefits.

5. Conclusions

While there are several reports that SA-containing ingredients may influence cognitive development, we found no evidence that bovine-derived dietary SL provided at 380 mg SL/L was effective at altering recognition memory or sleep-related activity.

Acknowledgments: The authors would like to thank Kristen Karkiewicz for her assistance with animal rearing. The authors acknowledge the efforts of Mead Johnson Nutrition employees Shireen Doultani and Julieta Ortiz for assistance in formulating and manufacturing the diets. The authors would also like to thank Monique LeBourgeois for her assistance with adapting actigraphy to the pig model and the Mead Johnson Nutrition Medical Affairs Department for donating the actigraphy devices.

Author Contributions: All authors contributed to design of the study. S.A.F. performed study execution. S.A.F. and R.N.D. contributed to statistical analyses. All authors contributed to interpretation and manuscript preparation.

Conflicts of Interest: The study was funded by Mead Johnson Nutrition, where Maciej Chichlowski is employed. Brian M. Berg was an employee of Mead Johnson Nutrition during study execution and manuscript preparation and Rhythm Pharmaceuticals at the time of publication. Sharon M. Donovan and Ryan N. Dilger have consulted for and received grant funding from Mead Johnson Nutrition.

References

1. Ballard, O.; Morrow, A.L. Human milk composition: Nutrients and bioactive factors. *Pediatr. Clin. N. Am.* **2013**, *60*, 49–74. [CrossRef] [PubMed]
2. Horta, B.L.; de Mola, C.L.; Victora, C.G. Breastfeeding and intelligence: A systematic review and meta-analysis. *Acta Paediatr. Int. J. Paediatr.* **2015**, *104*, 14–19. [CrossRef] [PubMed]
3. Girard, L.-C.; Doyle, O.; Tremblay, R.E. Breastfeeding, Cognitive and Noncognitive Development in Early Childhood: A Population Study. *Pediatrics* **2017**, *139*, e20161848. [CrossRef] [PubMed]
4. Hoffman, D.R.; Boettcher, J.A.; Diersen-Schade, D.A. Toward optimizing vision and cognition in term infants by dietary docosahexaenoic and arachidonic acid supplementation: A review of randomized controlled trials. *Prostaglandins Leukot. Essent. Fat. Acids* **2009**, *81*, 151–158. [CrossRef] [PubMed]
5. Zeisel, S.H. Nutritional Importance of Choline for Brain Development. *J. Am. Coll. Nutr.* **2004**, *23*, 621S–626S. [CrossRef] [PubMed]
6. Palmano, K.; Rowan, A.; Guillermo, R.; Guan, J.; McJarrow, P. The role of gangliosides in neurodevelopment. *Nutrients* **2015**, *7*, 3891–3913. [CrossRef] [PubMed]
7. Morrow, A.L.; Ruiz-Palacios, G.M.; Jiang, X.; Newburg, D.S. Human-milk glycans that inhibit pathogen binding protect breast-feeding infants against infectious diarrhea. *J. Nutr.* **2005**, *135*, 1304–1307. [CrossRef] [PubMed]
8. Bode, L. Human milk oligosaccharides: Every baby needs a sugar mama. *Glycobiology* **2012**, *22*, 1147–1162. [CrossRef] [PubMed]
9. Fleming, S.A.; Monaikul, S.; Patsavas, A.J.; Waworuntu, R.V.; Berg, B.M.; Dilger, R.N. Dietary polydextrose and galactooligosaccharide increase exploratory behavior, improve recognition memory, and alter neurochemistry in the young pig. *Nutr. Neurosci.* **2017**, 1–14. [CrossRef] [PubMed]
10. Vickers, M.H.; Guan, J.; Gustavsson, M.; Krägeloh, C.U.; Breier, B.H.; Davison, M.; Fong, B.; Norris, C.; McJarrow, P.; Hodgkinson, S.C. Supplementation with a mixture of complex lipids derived from milk to growing rats results in improvements in parameters related to growth and cognition. *Nutr. Res.* **2009**, *29*, 426–435. [CrossRef] [PubMed]
11. Liu, H.; Radlowski, E.E.C.; Conrad, M.M.S.; Li, Y.; Dilger, R.N.; Johnson, R.W. Early supplementation of phospholipids and gangliosides affects brain and cognitive development in neonatal piglets. *J. Nutr.* **2014**, *144*, 1–7. [CrossRef] [PubMed]
12. Wang, B.; Yu, B.; Karim, M.; Hu, H.; Sun, Y.; McGreevy, P.; Petocz, P.; Held, S.; Brand-Miller, J. Dietary sialic acid supplementation improves learning and memory in piglets. *Am. J. Clin. Nutr.* **2007**, *85*, 561–569. [CrossRef] [PubMed]
13. Chen, Y.; Zheng, Z.; Zhu, X.; Shi, Y.; Tian, D.; Zhao, F.; Liu, N.; Hüppi, P.S.; Troy, F.A.; Wang, B. Lactoferrin Promotes Early Neurodevelopment and Cognition in Postnatal Piglets by Upregulating the BDNF Signaling Pathway and Polysialylation. *Mol. Neurobiol.* **2015**, *52*, 256–269. [CrossRef] [PubMed]
14. Tarr, A.J.; Galley, J.D.; Fisher, S.E.; Chichlowski, M.; Berg, B.M.; Bailey, M.T. The prebiotics 3'Sialyllactose and 6'Sialyllactose diminish stressor-induced anxiety-like behavior and colonic microbiota alterations: Evidence for effects on the gut-brain axis. *Brain Behav. Immun.* **2015**, *50*, 166–177. [CrossRef] [PubMed]
15. Chichlowski, M.; Morairty, S.; Berg, B.M. Early life diet alters sleep architecture following an acute stress: The potential role of milk oligosaccharides. *FASEB J.* **2017**, *31*, 636.
16. Sakai, F.; Ikeuchi, Y.; Urashima, T.; Fujihara, M.; Ohtsuki, K.; Yanahira, S. Effects of Feeding Sialyllactose and Galactosylated *N*-Acetylneuraminic Acid on Swimming Learning Ability and Brain Lipid Composition in Adult Rats. *J. Appl. Glycosci.* **2006**, *53*, 249–254. [CrossRef]

17. Jacobi, S.K.; Yatsunenko, T.; Li, D.; Dasgupta, S.; Yu, R.K.; Berg, B.M.; Chichlowski, M.; Odle, J. Dietary Isomers of Sialyllactose Increase Ganglioside Sialic Acid Concentrations in the Corpus Callosum and Cerebellum and Modulate the Colonic Microbiota of Formula-Fed Piglets. *J. Nutr.* **2016**, *146*, 200–208. [PubMed]

18. Mudd, A.A.T.; Fleming, S.S.A.; Labhart, B.; Chichlowski, M.; Berg, B.B.M.; Donovan, S.S.M.; Dilger, R.R.N. Dietary Sialyllactose Influences Sialic Acid Concentrations in the Prefrontal Cortex and Magnetic Resonance Imaging Measures in Corpus Callosum of Young Pigs. *Nutrients* **2017**, *9*, 1297. [CrossRef] [PubMed]

19. Bruggencate, S.J.T.; Bovee-Oudenhoven, I.M.; Feitsma, A.L.; van Hoffen, E.; Schoterman, M.H. Functional role and mechanisms of sialyllactose and other sialylated milk oligosaccharides. *Nutr. Rev.* **2014**, *72*, 377–389. [CrossRef] [PubMed]

20. Fleming, S.A.; Dilger, R.N. Young pigs exhibit differential exploratory behavior during novelty preference tasks in response to age, sex, and delay. *Behav. Brain Res.* **2017**, *321*, 50–60. [CrossRef] [PubMed]

21. Martín-Sosa, S.; Martín, M.-J.; García-Pardo, L.A.; Hueso, P. Distribution of sialic acids in the milk of spanish mothers of full term infants during lactation. *J. Pediatr. Gastroenterol. Nutr.* **2004**, *39*, 499–503. [CrossRef] [PubMed]

22. Mudd, A.T.; Salcedo, J.; Alexander, L.S.; Johnson, S.K.; Getty, C.M.; Chichlowski, M.; Berg, B.M.; Barile, D.; Dilger, R.N. Porcine Milk Oligosaccharides and Sialic Acid Concentrations Vary throughout Lactation. *Front. Nutr.* **2016**, *3*. [CrossRef] [PubMed]

23. Spichtig, V.; Michaud, J.; Austin, S. Determination of sialic acids in milks and milk-based products. *Anal. Biochem.* **2010**, *405*, 28–40. [PubMed]

24. Röhrig, C.H.; Choi, S.S.H.; Baldwin, N. The nutritional role of free sialic acid, a human milk monosaccharide, and its application as a functional food ingredient. *Crit. Rev. Food Sci. Nutr.* **2017**, *57*, 1017–1038. [CrossRef] [PubMed]

25. Wang, B.; Hu, H.; Yu, B.; Troy, F.A. Molecular characterization of pig UDP-*N*-acetylglucosamine-2-epimerase/*N*-acetylmannosamine kinase (Gne) gene: Effect of dietary sialic acid supplementation on gene expression in piglets. *Curr. Top. Nutr. Res.* **2007**, *5*, 165–175.

26. Xu, X.; Zhu, T. Effect of ganglioside in repairing the neurological function of Chinese children with cerebral palsy. *Chin. J. Clin. Rehabil.* **2005**, *9*, 122–123.

27. Neelima; Sharma, R.; Rajput, Y.S.; Mann, B. Chemical and functional properties of glycomacropeptide (GMP) and its role in the detection of cheese whey adulteration in milk: A review. *Dairy Sci. Technol.* **2013**, *93*, 21–43. [CrossRef] [PubMed]

28. Levay, P.F.; Viljoen, M. Lactoferrin: A general review. *Haematologica* **1995**, *80*, 252–267. [PubMed]

29. Fagioli, S.; Rossi-Arnaud, C.; Castellano, C. Dose-dependent effect of GM1 ganglioside during development on inhibitory avoidance behaviour in mice: Influence of the period of administration. *Psychopharmacology (Berl.)* **1992**, *109*, 457–460. [CrossRef] [PubMed]

30. Silva, R.H.; Bellot, R.G.; Vital, M.A.; Frussa-Filho, R. Effects of long-term ganglioside GM1 administration on a new discriminative avoidance test in normal adult mice. *Psychopharmacology (Berl.)* **1997**, *129*, 322–328. [PubMed]

31. Fong, T.G.; Neff, N.H.; Hadjiconstantinou, M. GM1 ganglioside improves spatial learning and memory of aged rats. *Behav. Brain Res.* **1997**, *85*, 203–211. [CrossRef]

32. Silva, R.H.; Bergamo, M.; Frussa-Filho, R. Effects of neonatal ganglioside GM1 administration on memory in adult and old rats. *Pharmacol. Toxicol.* **2000**, *87*, 120–125. [CrossRef]

33. Popov, N.; Toffano, G.; Riechert, U.; Matthies, H. Effects of intraventricularly applied gangliosides and *N*-acetylneuraminic acid on acquisition and retention performance of a brightness discrimination task in rats. *Pharmacol. Biochem. Behav.* **1989**, *34*, 209–212. [CrossRef]

34. Silva, R.H.; Felicio, L.F.; Frussa-Filho, R. Ganglioside GM1 attenuates scopolamine-induced amnesia in rats and mice. *Psychopharmacology (Berl.)* **1999**, *141*, 111–117. [CrossRef] [PubMed]

35. Glasier, M.M.; Janis, L.S.; Goncalves, M.I.; Stein, D.G. GM1 produces attenuation of short-term memory deficits in Hebb-Williams maze performance after unilateral entorhinal cortex lesions. *Physiol. Behav.* **1999**, *66*, 441–446. [CrossRef]

36. Morgan, B.L.; Winick, M. Effects of administration of N-acetylneuraminic acid (NANA) on brain NANA content and behavior. *J. Nutr.* **1980**, *110*, 416–424. [CrossRef] [PubMed]

37. Wainwright, P.E.; Lomanowska, A.M.; McCutcheon, D.; Park, E.J.; Clandinin, M.T.; Ramanujam, K.S. Postnatal dietary supplementation with either gangliosides or choline: Effects on spatial short-term memory in artificially-reared rats. *Nutr. Neurosci.* **2007**, *10*, 67–77. [CrossRef] [PubMed]

38. Gustavsson, M.; Hodgkinson, S.C.; Fong, B.; Norris, C.; Guan, J.; Krageloh, C.U.; Breier, B.H.; Davison, M.; McJarrow, P.; Vickers, M.H. Maternal supplementation with a complex milk lipid mixture during pregnancy and lactation alters neonatal brain lipid composition but lacks effect on cognitive function in rats. *Nutr. Res.* **2010**, *30*, 279–289. [CrossRef] [PubMed]

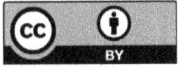

© 2018 by the authors. Licensee MDPI, Basel, Switzerland. This article is an open access article distributed under the terms and conditions of the Creative Commons Attribution (CC BY) license (http://creativecommons.org/licenses/by/4.0/).

nutrients

MDPI

Article

Effects of a Lutein and Zeaxanthin Intervention on Cognitive Function: A Randomized, Double-Masked, Placebo-Controlled Trial of Younger Healthy Adults

Lisa M. Renzi-Hammond [1,2], Emily R. Bovier [1,3], Laura M. Fletcher [1], L. Stephen Miller [1], Catherine M. Mewborn [1], Cutter A. Lindbergh [1], Jeffrey H. Baxter [4] and Billy R. Hammond Jr. [1,*]

[1]   Department of Psychology, The University of Georgia, Athens, GA 30602-3013, USA;
      lrenzi@uga.edu (L.M.R.-H.); emily.bovier@oswego.edu (E.R.B.); fletcher.lauram@gmail.com (L.M.F.);
      lsmiller@uga.edu (L.S.M.); mewborn@uga.edu (C.M.M.); cal@uga.edu (C.A.L.)
[2]   Institute of Gerontology, Department of Health Promotion and Behavior, College of Public Health,
      The University of Georgia, Athens, GA 30602, USA
[3]   Department of Psychology, State University of New York, Oswego Campus, Oswego, NY 13126, USA
[4]   Abbott Nutrition, Global Research and Development, Columbus, OH 43219, USA; jeffrey.baxter@abbott.com
*   Correspondence: bhammond@uga.edu; Tel.: +1-(706)-542-4812

Received: 28 September 2017; Accepted: 8 November 2017; Published: 14 November 2017

Abstract: Background: Past studies have suggested that higher lutein (L) and zeaxanthin (Z) levels in serum and in the central nervous system (as quantified by measuring macular pigment optical density, MPOD) are related to improved cognitive function in older adults. Very few studies have addressed the issue of xanthophylls and cognitive function in younger adults, and no controlled trials have been conducted to date to determine whether or not supplementation with L + Z can change cognitive function in this population. **Objective:** The purpose of this study was to determine whether or not supplementation with L + Z could improve cognitive function in young (age 18–30), healthy adults. **Design:** A randomized, double-masked, placebo-controlled trial design was used. Fifty-one young, healthy subjects were recruited as part of a larger study on xanthophylls and cognitive function. Subjects were randomized into active supplement ($n = 37$) and placebo groups ($n = 14$). MPOD was measured psychophysically using customized heterochromatic flicker photometry. Cognitive function was measured using the CNS Vital Signs testing platform. MPOD and cognitive function were measured every four months for a full year of supplementation. **Results:** Supplementation increased MPOD significantly over the course of the year, vs. placebo ($p < 0.001$). Daily supplementation with L + Z and increases in MPOD resulted in significant improvements in spatial memory ($p < 0.04$), reasoning ability ($p < 0.05$) and complex attention ($p < 0.04$), above and beyond improvements due to practice effects. **Conclusions:** Supplementation with L + Z improves CNS xanthophyll levels and cognitive function in young, healthy adults. Magnitudes of effects are similar to previous work reporting correlations between MPOD and cognition in other populations.

Keywords: xanthophylls; cognition; reasoning; visual memory; attention

---

1. Introduction

A wide body of research, across disciplines, has shown a direct effect of diet on nearly every aspect of brain function [1]. One big category of effect appears to be simply prophylactic. The brain is a strongly lipid-based, highly oxygenated structure prone to inflammatory stress. Dietary intake, good or bad, can influence the oxidative and inflammatory state of the brain and, hence, its function [2]. Another category is acute effects on cellular metabolism [3]. Dietary intake is involved in every aspect of a neuron's function, ranging from influencing the basic structure of the cell itself (e.g., phospholipid composition [4]); to resting and action potentials; to neurotransmitter synthesis from amino acid and vitamin precursors (e.g., pyridoxal 5′-phosphate, a form of Vitamin B_6, is a coenzyme required for the biosynthesis of gamma-aminobutyric acid (GABA), norepinephrine and serotonin from glutamic acid, tyrosine and tryptophan, respectively). B_6, B_{12} and folate are required to support methylation reactions, some of which are noted above, and are also important in gene regulation. It is interesting to note that methylation is the sole method for regulation of genes in mitochondrial DNA, and that these vitamins are critical for mitochondrial function.

Like many areas of nutrition, most research on the diet–brain connection has focused on micronutrient deficiencies, such as the role of B vitamins in cognitive decline or diseases such as Korsakoff's and dementia [5,6]. Much less is known about the many other phytochemicals that are commonly found in food (i.e., not yet defined as essential or even as nutrients). Even less is known about how those components of diet influence the brains of young healthy adults. One exception to this general trend is a growing interest in a possible role for the xanthophylls, specifically lutein (L), zeaxanthin (Z) and meso-zeaxanthin (MZ) [7]. These dietary carotenoids concentrate in neural tissue (particularly, the macula or central retina, there termed macular pigment (MP)). Unlike many dietary components, the amount of retinal L, Z and MZ can be measured directly and non-invasively [8]. MPOD has been shown to be highly correlated to L + Z accumulation in brain [9]. This allows the concentration of these xanthophylls in neural tissue to be correlated with dependent measures of interest. Using this technique, a number of cross-sectional studies have correlated the macular xanthophylls with many aspects of both visual and cognitive function in both young and older subjects [10–15].

The ability to directly measure the macular pigments also provides the additional advantage of being able to monitor the results of an intervention; to wit, one can supplement L, Z or MZ, measure changes in MP, and then assess any possible functional changes that result (and how those changes relate to the actual change in tissue levels). Using this strategy, a number of studies have now shown that supplementing L and Z is related to both increases in the amount of L + Z measured in the retina and alteration in behaviors that are thought to be primarily mediated by the brain. For example, supplementation with carotenoid-rich avocados causes increases in both the macular pigments and spatial working memory [16]. This improvement was not found for control subjects whose carotenoid levels did not increase. L + Z supplementation in healthy older adults produces improvements in cognitive function on a variety of domains [17–19]. Such effects have even been found in young healthy subjects (i.e., those seemingly less likely to change). For example, Bovier et al. [14,15] supplemented young subjects and found changes in visual temporal processing speed in subjects whose MP increased by 0.1 log units of optical density or more, versus those that did not, using a placebo-controlled design. Visual processing speed was chosen because, although it is a lower level visual function (basically, the fusion of square-and sine wave modulated light), it is thought to be mediated by central brain mechanisms (e.g., [20]). Indeed, some have argued that processing speed in general underlies many more complex cognitive traits [21] and should be considered a cognitive fundamental [22]. The results by Bovier et al. implied the possibility that supplementing xanthophylls could change other aspects of cognition (such as memory) even in young healthy subjects at the (apparent) peak of their cognitive life (e.g., college students). The present study was a first test of this hypothesis.

2. Materials and Methods

2.1. Subjects

This sub-study was part of a larger clinical trial on xanthophyll supplementation and cognitive function. For the young adult sub-study, a total of 79 potential participants (college students from the Athens-Clarke County, GA area) were screened for enrollment between August 2012 and December 2013, with follow-up lasting through December 2014. Of those 79 potential participants, three participants were initially excluded for failure to meet the inclusion criteria.

Randomization to either the active supplement group or the placebo group was accomplished as follows: a set of numerical codes was created that corresponded to either the active supplement or the intervention. The codes were placed into an opaque envelope. After informed consent was signed and inclusion/exclusion criteria were verified (see below), a code was drawn from the envelope by the clinical coordinator, who had no data collection responsibilities. From the 76 participants who were deemed eligible for participation, 30 participants were randomized into the placebo group, and 46 total participants were randomized into the intervention group. Of those participants, two members of the placebo group and three members of the intervention group withdrew from the trial due to scheduling conflicts prior to completion of baseline measurements and allocation of supplements. Given the fact that students enrolled in the trial occasionally graduated and moved away during the study, 14 total placebo participants and 9 total intervention participants were lost to follow-up during the course of the year-long intervention.

The final analyzable data set included 51 healthy subjects ranging in age from 18 to 30 ($M = 21.21 \pm 2.52$) years. Approximately equal numbers of males and females ($n = 29$ males, 22 females) were analyzed, with a total of $n = 14$ participants in the placebo group, and $n = 37$ participants who received the intervention. The active supplement contained 10 mg L + 2 mg Z (DSM Nutritional Products; Kaiseraugst, Switzerland), and the placebo was visually identical to the active supplement. Supplement and placebo containers were visually identical, with the exception of the numerical code on the bottle contents label. Participants were instructed to take one tablet per day with their highest fat meal. Compliance with the supplement regime was monitored by bi-monthly phone calls as well as pill counts.

The baseline characteristics of the entire analyzable young adult sample, as well as the two sub-groups, are shown in Table 1. The majority of the subjects were students from the University of Georgia, and placebo and active supplement groups were not significantly different from each other in demographic characteristics. Inclusion criteria included good overall and ocular/refractive (20:40 best corrected acuity) health and no supplement use in the previous six months (excluding a multivitamin containing less than 1 mg LZ/day).

Table 1. Baseline characteristics of placebo participants vs. those on the active supplement.

Group	Age (Years)	Body Mass Index	Gender	Ethnicity	Race	Years of Education	MP Optical Density
Active, Mean ± SD	21.50 ± 2.69	24.15 ± 3.86	21 M, 16 F	$n = 35$ non-Hispanic $n = 2$ Hispanic	$n = 30$ White $n = 4$ Black $n = 1$ pan-Asian $n = 2$ Latino	12+	0.47 ± 0.18
Placebo, Mean ± SD	20.50 ± 1.91	23.03 ± 3.98	8 M, 6 F	$n = 14$ non-Hispanic	$n = 10$ White $n = 2$ Black $n = 2$ pan-Asian	12+	0.39 ± 0.12

None of the differences between the groups were statistically significant at baseline ($p > 0.05$). SD = standard deviation. M = male; F = female.

2.2. Ethics

The tenets of the Declaration of Helsinki were adhered to at all times during the course of this study. All participants both verbally consented to participation and provided written informed consent prior to participation. The protocol was approved by the University of Georgia Institutional Review Board (2012105172).

2.3. Methods

2.3.1. Retinal L + Z Levels

Retinal L + Z levels (as macular pigment optical density, MPOD) was measured at 30-min of retinal eccentricity along the horizontal meridian of the temporal retina, using customized heterochromatic flicker photometry (cHFP) [23,24]. Briefly, a macular densitometer (Macular Metrics; Rehoboth, MA, USA) was used to present participants with a one-degree test stimulus composed of light generated by two narrow-band LEDs, peaking at 460 nm (strongly absorbed by MP) and 570 nm (not absorbed by MP), respectively. Each waveband was presented in counter-phase orientation at two different starting intensities, which, when combined, appeared to participants as a single, uniform, flickering disk. The stimulus was presented on a 470 nm background.

Participants were required to centrally view the stimulus, and to adjust the intensity of the 460 nm test light relative to the 570 nm reference light until the appearance of flicker was minimized. The participants then viewed a larger (two-degree) stimulus while fixating on a point at 7-degrees of retinal eccentricity. This placed the stimulus on the parafovea, where MPOD is negligible. Participants completed five trials at each locus. The two loci were compared to yield MPOD at 30-min of eccentricity. MPOD was measured at baseline, and after 4-, 8- and 12-month supplementation.

2.3.2. Serum L + Z Levels

In addition to measuring CNS L + Z levels (as MPOD), L + Z were measured in the serum via high performance liquid chromatography (HPLC) to confirm participant compliance. The methods used to collect serum samples and measure L and Z concentration have been presented previously [25].

2.3.3. Cognitive Function

Cognitive function was tested using a computerized test battery (CNS Vital Signs; Morrisville, NC, USA) at baseline, 4-, 8- and 12-month time points [26]. The procedure used to collect cognitive function data was presented previously [18]. Briefly, in order to complete computerized tests, participants were seated in front of a Dell E 2211H 18-inch monitor with a full QWERTY keyboard. A research assistant familiar with the test procedure remained in the room with the participant during the entire test protocol. Visual acuity of 20:40 or better was confirmed prior to enrollment. Prior to each test set, participants were given a practice session to confirm that test instructions were clear.

Individual functional tests and cognitive domains computed by raw scores on these tests are listed in Table 2, and have been presented previously [18]. During the test session, participants were given the same sequence of individual tests, each designed to measure some aspect of cognitive function. Raw scores on these individual tests were used to calculate cognitive domain scores, which were used in statistical analysis. For example, average numbers of taps executed by the right and left hands on the Finger Tapping Test were combined with the number of correct responses on the Symbol-Digit Coding task to compute the Psychomotor Speed domain score. Errors on the Stroop Task, Continuous Performance Task and Shifting Attention Task were combined to compute the Complex Attention domain score. For a complete list of tests administered, domains computed and computation parameters, see Table 2 and [18].

Table 2. Individual tests administered and cognitive domains evaluated in the test battery.

Domain	Corresponding Tests	Computation Procedure
Verbal Memory (VeM)	Verbal Memory Test	Correct hits for presented words + correct passes on distractors for tests immediately after presentation and after a 30-min delay.
Visual Memory (ViM)	Visual Memory Test	Correct hits for presented shapes and symbols + correct passes on distractors for tests immediately after presentation and after a 30-min delay.
Reasoning (R)	Non-Verbal Reasoning Test (NVRT)	Correct responses on the NVRT − commission errors on the NVRT.
Executive Function (EF)	Shifting Attention Test (SAT)	Correct responses on the SAT − errors on the SAT.

Table 2. *Cont.*

Domain	Corresponding Tests	Computation Procedure
Psychomotor Speed (PmS)	Finger Tapping Test (FTT) Symbol-Digit Coding Test (SDC)	Average number of taps on the FTT with the right hand + average number of taps with the left hand + number of correct responses on the SDC
Complex Attention (CA)	Stroop Test (ST) SAT Continuous Performance Task (CPT)	Commission errors on the ST + Errors on the SAT + Commission and omission errors on the CPT
Cognitive Flexibility (CF)	SAT ST	Correct responses on the SAT − errors on the SAT − Commission errors on the ST

Note: Raw scores computed as described above were used in all statistical analyses.

2.3.4. Statistical Analyses and other Considerations

All statistical analyses were performed using SPSS version 23 (IBM) with $p < 0.05$ as the criterion for significance. The following domain scores were compared in statistical analyses: verbal memory, visual memory, reasoning, executive function, psychomotor speed, complex attention and cognitive flexibility. All tests were one-tailed, given the directional nature of the a priori hypotheses, specified below. The relationship between nutritional status and cognitive function was analyzed in two ways, as follows:

First, domain scores from participants on the placebo were directly compared against domain scores from participants taking the active supplement. To make these comparisons, difference scores were computed between baseline and 12-month time points for each cognitive domain tested, and those difference scores were compared between groups receiving placebo and those receiving the active supplement, for each domain. This comparison tests whether or not supplementation with L + Z was able to improve MPOD (the study biomarker of CNS xanthophyll levels) and whether such increases could affect cognitive function.

The second set of comparisons was aimed at addressing two major issues commonly seen in nutritional trials: poor compliance and dietary change. Non-compliance with the study regimen is seen in a number of clinical trials, from drug trials to nutrition trials, and we expected that some participants would not consistently take their nutritional supplement. Those in the active group who did not consistently take their supplements would, we predicted, have performance similar to placebo participants, rather than to other active supplement users.

The issue of dietary change is more complex. Although many nutrition trials (this trial included) are double-masked, to adhere to the tenets of the Declaration of Helsinki, participants should to the extent possible be informed about the nature of the trial. This model is most commonly used in drug trials, where participants either cannot acquire or would have some difficulty acquiring the active agent being tested. In nutrition trials that follow this "gold standard" randomized, double-masked, placebo-controlled trial model, once participants know the identity of the test supplement and the motivation for testing it, they can do individual research on the ingredients within that supplement and actually acquire the test molecules via the diet (or, if available, as is true in this case, in supplement form). In the current study, for example, participants were told at baseline that they would be taking either an active supplement containing L + Z or a visually identical placebo to examine putative benefits of these molecules on cognitive function. Given that fact, we expected that participants who researched the foods that naturally contain L and Z to learn more about the molecules might (even unintentionally) start increasing intakes of L- and Z-containing foods. For placebo group participants, we predicted that these dietary changes (or the frank obtaining of actives in the dietary supplement market) would cause performance to look more like the performance of active supplement users. Finally, it is well known that participants in clinical trials with diet questionnaires will unconsciously improve their diet (and in some cases other aspects of their lifestyle (exercise, alcohol intake and so forth) over the course of the study—perhaps simply because they know someone is "watching".

In an attempt to determine whether or not participants changed dietary intakes, a food frequency questionnaire (FFQ) was collected at baseline and 12-month time points to measure fruit and vegetable intake. Participants in both groups tended to slightly increase the number of servings of fruits and vegetables consumed per day between baseline (3+ servings of fruits + vegetables per day) and 12 months (4+ servings/day). With respect to the compliance issue, compliance calls, pill counts and serum analysis suggested that 6 out of 37 participants in the active group were not fully compliant over the course of the year with the supplement regiment (these participants reported forgetting to take pills in at least three compliance phone calls), and thus would be less likely to show changes in MP optical density, the study biomarker of increased L + Z levels in the CNS. Finally, past research [27] has suggested that a small subset of the population is likely unable to absorb and/or appropriately traffic L and Z, and thus would not show serum and retinal responses even if they were fully compliant with the supplementation regimen.

To address these issues statistically, difference scores between MPOD at baseline and 12 months were computed. All participants who showed an increase of 0.10+ log units of MPOD, regardless of randomized group membership at study entry, were then grouped ($n = 27$) and were compared against participants whose MPOD did not increase ($n = 24$). Cognitive performance was then compared between those whose MPOD increased vs. those who did not increase. This comparison indicates whether or not increases in CNS L + Z (as predicted by MPOD measures) can improve cognitive function, irrespective of what caused the increased L + Z status.

3. Results

3.1. Retinal L + Z Levels

At baseline, MPOD in the study sample was higher ($M = 0.48 \pm 0.18$) than previously published averages for healthy adults (M = approximately 0.3; [28,29]), indicating that the sample was relatively well-nourished. Following one year of supplementation, those on the active supplement increased significantly ($p < 0.001$) between the baseline ($M = 0.47 \pm 0.18$) and 12-month ($M = 0.56 \pm 0.16$) time-points. The participants on placebo did not increase significantly (baseline: 0.40 ± 0.12, 12-month: 0.44 ± 0.18; $p > 0.05$).

3.2. Serum L + Z Levels

At baseline, serum L, Z and L + Z levels were not significantly different between the participants randomized into the active supplement group vs. the placebo group (see Table 3). Following one year of supplementation, serum L ($p = 0.029$), Z ($p = 0.011$) and L + Z ($p = 0.023$) levels were all significantly higher in the active supplement group than the placebo group (see Table 4, Figure 1).

Table 3. Baseline serum levels by supplement group.

Group	Serum Lutein (ng/µL)	Serum Zeaxanthin (ng/µL)	Lutein + Zeaxanthin (ng/µL)
Active, Mean ± SD	0.11 ± 0.07	0.03 ± 0.02	0.14 ± 0.08
Placebo, Mean ± SD	0.10 ± 0.03	0.03 ± 0.02	0.13 ± 0.04

None of the differences between the groups were statistically significant at baseline.

Table 4. Serum levels following one year of supplementation.

Group	Serum Lutein (ng/µL)	Serum Zeaxanthin (ng/µL)	Lutein + Zeaxanthin (ng/µL)
Active, Mean ± SD	0.38 ± 0.28	0.08 ± 0.05	0.46 ± 0.32
Placebo, Mean ± SD	0.19 ± 0.19	0.04 ± 0.04	0.23 ± 0.23

Note: Statistically significant differences were seen between the placebo group and the control group for serum L (p = 0.029), Z (p = 0.011), and L + Z (p = 0.023) following one year of supplementation.

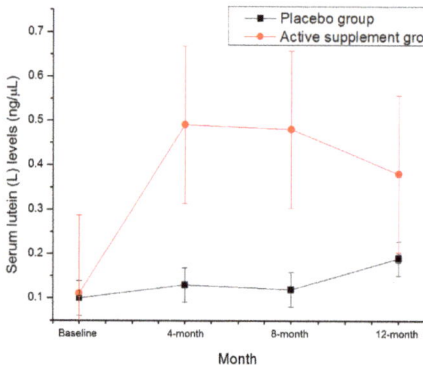

(**a**) Serum L changes across time.

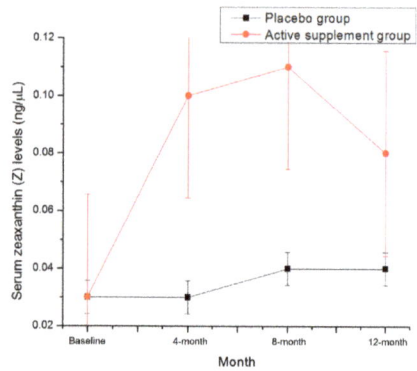

(**b**) Serum Z changes across time.

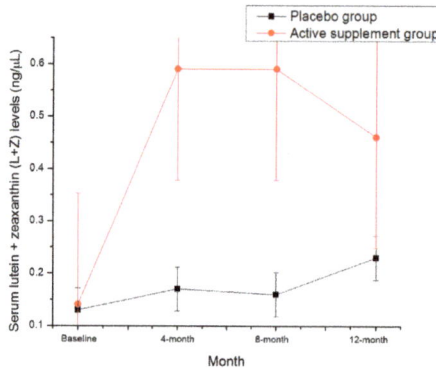

(**c**) Combined serum L + Z changes over time.

Figure 1. Serum changes from baseline to 12-month time points in: (**a**) lutein (L); (**b**) zeaxanthin (Z); and (**c**) and lutein + zeaxanthin (L + Z). Error bars represent the standard deviation of the mean at each time point.

3.3. Cognitive Function

At baseline, participants were not significantly different from each other on any of the cognitive domains tested. Given the fact that participants were tested four times throughout the course of the study, practice effects were anticipated, and seen, regardless of group identity (see Table 5).

As mentioned previously, not all members of the supplement group were compliant with the intervention, and some of the members of the placebo group also had increases in MPOD (likely due to dietary changes since the intervention was an entire year). Consequently, analyses were conducted in two ways: by supplement group, and by percent increase in MPOD, regardless of group membership. With respect to supplement status, after 12 months of supplementation, participants taking the active supplement had significantly higher performance on visual memory tasks ($p < 0.04$) than those participants taking the placebo (see Figure 2). Analysis of the Reliable Change Index (RCI) using a standard criterion of 1.96 for both groups suggested that the effects seen in the active supplement group were not simply due to practice effects (RCI active = 6.77; RCI placebo = 1.88).

Table 5. Practice effects demonstrated by improvement in cognitive function across domains, regardless of supplementation status.

Group	Verbal Memory	Visual Memory	Reasoning Ability	Executive Function	Complex Attention *	Cognitive Flexibility
Baseline Mean, all subjects	54.22	41.04	9.06	53.73	7.38	52.02
12-Month Mean, all subjects	56.26	49.24	10.20	62.59	5.98	60.65
Average change between baseline and 12 months, placebo group participants	3.57	4.93	1.64	8.86	0.46	8.43

* Lower score = fewer errors; for all other scores, an increase indicates improved performance.

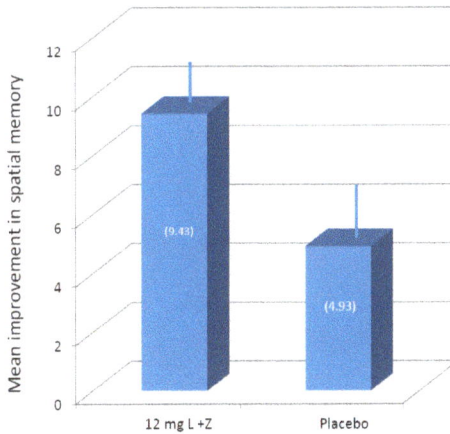

Figure 2. Average (with standard error of the mean, SEM) improvement in spatial memory following one-year supplementation. L, lutein; Z, zeaxanthin.

With respect to percent increase in MPOD, baseline MPOD was subtracted from 12-month MPOD scores. Participants who had numerical increases of 0.10 or greater were classified as "increasers", and participants who did not increase by a minimum of 0.10 were classified as "flat liners", regardless of supplement group assignment. Compared to "flat liners", participants with improvements of at least 0.10 for MPOD not only maintained significant differences in visual memory ($p < 0.05$) also scored significantly higher in the complex attention ($p < 0.04$) and reasoning ability ($p < 0.05$) tasks (see Figures 3 and 4). Analysis of the RCIs for each task suggested, again, that the differences seen in complex attention (RCI for "increasers" = 2.02; RCI for "flat liners" = 0.00) and likely reasoning ability (RCI for "increasers" = 1.94; RCI for "flat liners" = 0.18) were not due simply to practice effects.

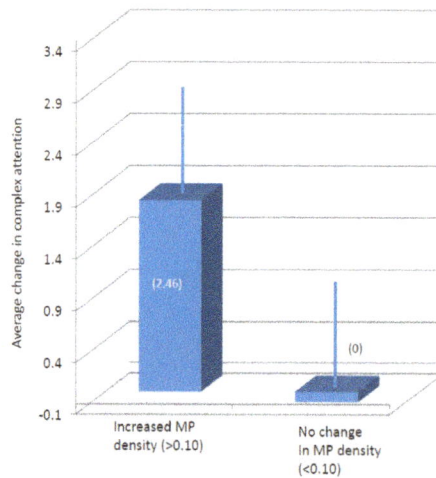

Figure 3. Average (and standard error of the mean (SEM)) change in complex attention segregated according to changes in macular pigment (MP) density.

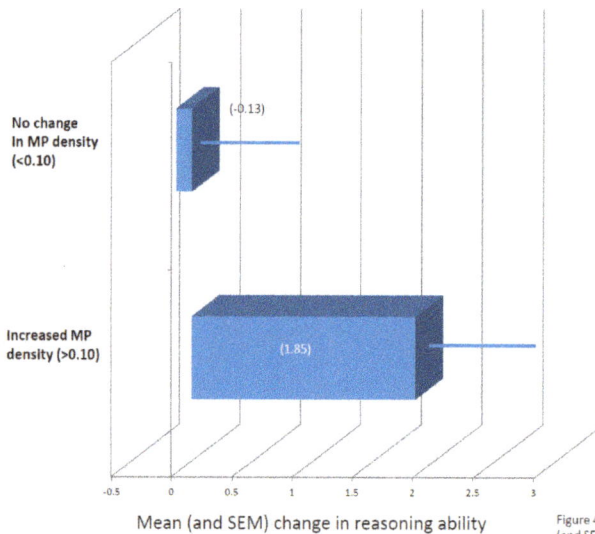

Mean (and SEM) change in reasoning ability

Figure 4. Average change (and SEM) of subjects whose MP changed and did not change

Figure 4. Average change (and SEM) of subjects whose MP changed and did not change.

4. Discussion

This randomized, double-masked, placebo-controlled study tested the effects of one year of nutritional supplementation (10 mg of L and 2 mg of Z) on the cognitive function of healthy, well-nourished college students. L and Z were picked because they are commonly available in supplement form (often marketed for eye health) and the xanthophylls are commonly found in food (e.g., supplementing spinach will directly increase retinal levels [27]). They can also be easily measured in central nervous tissue (neural retina) [8] and are found in some key locations in the brain, such as hippocampus, and frontal and occipital cortex [9]. We originally speculated that changing cognitive function via a simple dietary intervention in young well-nourished college students was unlikely. Past studies, such as the companion older adult sample tested in the larger study from which these data were drawn [18], and others (e.g., [19]) have shown improvements in cognitive function in older adults. Older adult samples tend to have baseline cognitive function that is more variable (e.g., [10,11,13]), with a higher proportion of individuals who are at risk for dementia. Consequently, the older adult population is likely to an easier population in which to demonstrate change. This young adult, highly educated sample was selected deliberately to isolate treatment effects that were not likely to be confounded by education status, underlying nutritional deficiency, or progression toward cognitive impairment. Nonetheless, we were able to measure several distinct cognitive benefits that were directly tied to increasing central nervous system levels of L and Z, as shown by increased MPOD, even though the starting MPOD levels were substantially higher than those previously reported for the general population.

The most significant effect according to treatment was visual memory: the treated group changed but the placebos did not. In a recent study that tested retinal and brain L and Z levels in human decedents, L tended to be relatively highly concentrated in occipital cortex, and L + Z levels in neural retina tended to be highly ($r = 0.78$) correlated to brain levels of the macular carotenoids in occipital lobe [9]. This current study represents the first of its kind that suggests that increasing CNS L + Z can also improve performance in a function that is mediated in large part by occipital cortex, which preferentially accumulates L + Z relative to the other carotenoids more commonly consumed in the diet [30] in young, otherwise healthy, high performing subjects.

Visual memory is a relatively low-level cognitive function. Sometimes referred to as stimulus memory [31], it reflects dynamic cortical changes resulting from the storage or processing of visual stimuli. It is the stage that precedes processing by other structures such as the hippocampus which encodes more complex visual memories such as maps or scenes. Visual memory is hard to distinguish from attention since some aspects of the stimulus must be attended to in order to enter visual memory in the first place [32]. Characteristics such as visual memory, attention and processing speed have all, in turn, been related to improved reasoning ability [22,33].

In our study, the xanthophyll intervention was related to all three of these variables: visual memory, complex attention and reasoning ability. Specifically, improved visual memory was related to the treatment; complex attention and reasoning ability were improved only if significant increases in MP were also achieved. The fact that L + Z supplementation was related specifically to these variables in the younger adults may not be coincidence. As noted, these three cognitive functions are, in some ways, related to each other. Our results further suggest, however, that they are physiologically connected in a way that xanthophylls could improve, even in the young, who are, theoretically, also near ceiling in these functions. Earlier data from our lab has indicated that speed of processing in young subjects can also be changed by changing MPOD [14,15]. It is important to note that the intervention was not related to change in any of the other cognitive functions tested, and some of the functions that improved in the companion older adult sample [18] did not also improve in the young adult sample. Additional neuroimaging analyses of the entire study sample, including the older adult sample, suggests that L + Z supplementation improves white matter integrity in regions of brain known to show white matter declines in older age, and in those at risk for dementia [34]. Supplementation with L + Z also buffers against age-related declines in verbal learning and memory and improves cerebral perfusion in older adults [17]. Consequently, L + Z might be serving multiple functions in the CNS, some of which are more important in older age.

One common factor that could affect all of these functions is a general improvement in neural efficiency, a hypothesis proposed for L + Z in 2010 [35]. Hence, increasing central levels of L + Z could improve neural efficiency, which would both speed neural conduction while simultaneously reducing the likelihood of cross-talk between axons. Such basic effects can influence higher functions. The latter, for instance, could lower interference allowing multiple representations within the brain

Nutrients **2017**, *9*, 1246

to be maintained and operated upon. We are currently using neuroimaging methods to assess these possibilities.

In the current study, several limitations should be considered with respect to generalizability. As mentioned previously, this sample was selected with the intention of avoiding both underlying nutritional deficiency that can contribute to poor cognitive performance, and cognitive differences between subjects that are due to differences in education level. Consequently, we ended up with a sample that should have been difficult to improve. The fact that these participants were well-nourished and cognitively high performing at baseline may limit generalizability to those with, for example, cognitive and neurological disease states.

Acknowledgments: The authors would like to acknowledge Matthew Tankersley and Medina Bello for their assistance with study coordination and data management, and Joanne Curran-Celentano and Karen Semo for assistance with serum analysis. This work was supported by Abbott Nutrition; Columbus, OH. Active supplements and placebos were supplied by DSM Nutritional Products; Basel, Switzerland.

Author Contributions: L.M.R.-H., B.R.H. and L.S.M. contributed to research study design; L.M.R.-H., B.R.H., E.R.B., L.M.F., L.S.M., C.M.M. and C.A.L. collected study data; J.H.B. provided study materials; L.M.R.-H., B.R.H. and L.S.M. contributed to data analysis; L.M.R.-H. and B.R.H. drafted the initial manuscript; L.M.R.-H., B.R.H., J.H.B. and L.S.M. primarily edited the manuscript; and L.M.R.-H., E.R.B., L.M.F., L.S.M., J.H.B., C.A.L., C.M.M. and B.R.H. assume responsibility for the final content of the manuscript.

Conflicts of Interest: Authors L.M.R.-H. and B.R.H. have received honoraria from Abbott Nutrition for presentation of research findings and L.R.H. was employed by Abbott Nutrition for a portion of the data collection period. Author J.H.B. was an employee of Abbott Nutrition. No other authors have conflicts of interest to disclose.

Registry Information: ClinicalTrials.gov number, NCT02023645.

Abbreviations

L	lutein
Z	zeaxanthin
MPOD	macular pigment optical density
MZ	meso-zeaxanthin
CNS	central nervous system
MP	macular pigment
HPLC	high-performance liquid chromatography
FFQ	food frequency questionnaire
RCI	reliable change index
VeM	verbal memory
ViM	visual memory
R	reasoning
EF	executive function
PmS	psychomotor speed
CA	complex attention
CF	cognitive flexibility
NVRT	non-verbal reasoning test
SAT	shifting attention test
FTT	finger tapping test
SDC	symbol-digit coding
ST	Stroop test
CPT	continuous performance task

References

1. Gomez-Pinilla, F. Brain foods: The effects of nutrients on brain function. *Nat. Rev. Neurosci.* **2008**, *9*, 568–578. [CrossRef] [PubMed]
2. Joseph, J.A.; Shukitt-Hale, B.; Casadesus, G.; Fisher, D. Oxidative stress and inflammation in brain aging: Nutritional considerations. *Neurochem. Res.* **2005**, *30*, 927–935. [CrossRef] [PubMed]

3. Bourre, J.M. Effects of nutrients (in food) on the structure and function of the nervous system: Update on dietary requirements for brain. Part 1: Micronutrients. *J. Nutr. Health Aging* **2006**, *10*, 377–385. [PubMed]

4. Carlson, S.E.; Carver, J.D.; House, S.G. High fat diets varying in ratios of polyunsaturated to saturated fatty acid and linoleic to linolenic acid: A comparison of rat neural and red cell membrane phospholipids. *J. Nutr.* **1986**, *116*, 718–725. [PubMed]

5. Cook, C.C.; Thomson, A.D. B-complex vitamins in the prophylaxis and treatment of Wernicke-Korsakoff syndrome. *Br. J. Hosp. Med.* **1997**, *57*, 461–465. [PubMed]

6. McCaddon, A.; Regland, B.; Hudson, P.; Davies, G. Functional vitamin B12 deficiency and Alzheimer disease. *Neurology* **2002**, *58*, 1395–1399. [CrossRef] [PubMed]

7. Erdman, J.W.; Smith, J.W.; Kuchan, M.J.; Mohn, E.S.; Johnson, E.J.; Rubakhin, S.S.; Wang, L.; Sweedler, J.V.; Neuringer, M. Lutein and Brain Function. *Foods* **2015**, *4*, 547–564. [CrossRef] [PubMed]

8. Hammond, B.R.J.; Wooten, B.R.; Smollon, B. Assessment of the validity of in vivo methods of measuring human macular pigment optical density. *Optom. Vis. Sci.* **2005**, *82*, 387–404. [CrossRef] [PubMed]

9. Vishwanathan, R.; Schalch, W.; Johnson, E.J. Macular pigment carotenoids in the retina and occipital cortex are related in humans. *Nutr. Neurosci.* **2015**, *19*, 95–101. [CrossRef] [PubMed]

10. Renzi, L.M.; Dengler, M.J.; Puente, A.; Miller, L.S.; Hammond, B.R.J. Relationships between macular pigment optical density and cognitive function in unimpaired and mildly cognitively impaired older adults. *Neurobiol. Aging* **2014**, *35*, 1695–1699. [CrossRef] [PubMed]

11. Feeney, J.; Finucane, C.; Savva, G.M.; Cronin, H.; Beatty, S.; Nolan, J.M.; Kenny, R.A. Low macular pigment optical density is associated with lower cognitive performance in a large, population-based sample of older adults. *Neurobiol. Aging* **2013**, *34*, 2449–2456. [CrossRef] [PubMed]

12. Kelly, D.; Coen, R.F.; Akuffo, K.O.; Beatty, S.; Dennison, J.; Moran, R.; Stack, J.; Howard, A.N.; Mulcahy, R.; Nolan, J.M. Cognitive Function and Its Relationship with Macular Pigment Optical Density and Serum Concentrations of its Constituent Carotenoids. *J. Alzheimers Dis.* **2015**, *48*, 261–277. [CrossRef] [PubMed]

13. Vishwanathan, R.; Iannaccone, A.; Scott, T.M.; Kritchevsky, S.B.; Jennings, B.J.; Carboni, G.; Forma, G.; Satterfield, S.; Harris, T.; Johnson, K.C.; et al. Macular pigment optical density is related to cognitive function in older people. *Age Ageing* **2014**, *43*, 271–275. [CrossRef] [PubMed]

14. Bovier, E.R.; Renzi, L.M.; Hammond, B.R. A double-blind, placebo-controlled study on the effects of lutein and zeaxanthin on neural processing speed and efficiency. *PLoS ONE* **2014**, *9*, e108178. [CrossRef] [PubMed]

15. Bovier, E.R.; Hammond, B.R. A randomized placebo-controlled study on the effects of lutein and zeaxanthin on visual processing speed in young healthy subjects. *Arch. Biochem. Biophys.* **2015**, *572*, 54–57. [CrossRef] [PubMed]

16. Johnson, E.; Vishwanathan, R.; Mohn, E.; Haddock, J.; Rasmussen, H.; Scott, T. Avocado Consumption Increases Neural Lutein and Improves Cognitive Function. *FASEB J.* **2015**, *29*, 32.8.

17. Lindbergh, C.A.; Renzi-Hammond, L.M.; Hammond, B.R.; Terry, D.P.; Mewborn, C.M.; Puente, A.N.; Miller, L.S. Lutein and Zeaxanthin Influence Brain Function in Older Adults: A Randomized Controlled Trial. *J. Int. Neuropsychol. Soc.* **2017**, 1–14. [CrossRef] [PubMed]

18. Hammond, B.R.; Miller, L.S.; Bello, M.O.; Lindbergh, C.A.; Mewborn, C.; Renzi-Hammond, L.M. Effects of Lutein/Zeaxanthin Supplementation on the Cognitive Function of Community Dwelling Older Adults: A Randomized, Double-Masked, Placebo-Controlled Trial. *Front. Aging Neurosci.* **2017**, *9*, 254. [CrossRef] [PubMed]

19. Johnson, E.J.; McDonald, K.; Caldarella, S.M.; Chung, H.-Y.; Troen, A.M.; Snodderly, D.M. Cognitive findings of an exploratory trial of docosahexaenoic acid and lutein supplementation in older women. *Nutr. Neurosci.* **2008**, *11*, 75–83. [CrossRef] [PubMed]

20. Zlody, R.L. The Relationship between Critical Flicker Frequency (CFF) and Several Intellectual Measures. *Am. J. Psychol.* **1965**, *78*, 596. [CrossRef] [PubMed]

21. Owsley, C. Visual processing speed. *Vis. Res.* **2013**, *90*, 52–56. [CrossRef] [PubMed]

22. Satlhouse, D.J.; Timothy, A.; Madden, D.J. Information Processing Speed and Aging. In *Information Processing Speed in Clinical Populations*; DeLuca, J., Kalmar, J.H., Eds.; Taylor and Frances: New York, NY, USA, 2008; pp. 221–242.

23. Stringham, J.M.; Hammond, B.R.; Nolan, J.M.; Wooten, B.R.; Mammen, A.; Smollon, W.; Snodderly, D.M. The utility of using customized heterochromatic flicker photometry (cHFP) to measure macular pigment in patients with age-related macular degeneration. *Exp. Eye Res.* **2008**, *87*, 445–453. [CrossRef] [PubMed]

24. Wooten, B.R.; Hammond, B.R.; Land, R.I.; Snodderly, D.M. A practical method for measuring macular pigment optical density. *Investig. Ophthalmol. Vis. Sci.* **1999**, *40*, 2481–2489.

25. Lindbergh, C.A.; Mewborn, C.M.; Hammond, B.R.; Renzi-Hammond, L.M.; Curran-Celentano, J.M.; Miller, L.S. Relationship of Lutein and Zeaxanthin Levels to Neurocognitive Functioning: An fMRI Study of Older Adults. *J. Int. Neuropsychol. Soc.* **2017**, *23*, 11–22. [CrossRef] [PubMed]

26. Gualtieri, C.T.; Johnson, L.G. Reliability and validity of a computerized neurocognitive test battery, CNS Vital Signs. *Arch. Clin. Neuropsychol.* **2006**, *21*, 623–643. [CrossRef] [PubMed]

27. Hammond, B.R., Jr.; Johnson, E.J.; Russell, R.M.; Krinsky, N.I.; Yeum, K.J.; Edwards, R.B.; Snodderly, D.M. Dietary modification of human macular pigment density. *Investig. Ophthalmol. Vis. Sci.* **1997**, *38*, 1795–1801.

28. Hammond, B.R.; Caruso-Avery, M. Macular pigment optical density in a Southwestern sample. *Investig. Ophthalmol. Vis. Sci.* **2000**, *41*, 1492–1497.

29. Curran-Celentano, J.; Hammond, B.R.; Ciulla, T.A.; Cooper, D.A.; Pratt, L.M.; Danis, R.B. Relation between dietary intake, serum concentrations, and retinal concentrations of lutein and zeaxanthin in adults in a Midwest population. *Am. J. Clin. Nutr.* **2001**, *74*, 796–802. [PubMed]

30. Craft, N.; Dorey, C.K. Carotenoid, tocopherol, and retinal concentrations in elderly human brain. *J. Nutr. Health Aging* **2004**, *8*, 156–162. [PubMed]

31. Murray, E.A. What have ablation studies told us about the neural substrates of stimulus memory? *Semin. Neurosci.* **1996**, *8*, 13–22. [CrossRef]

32. Downing, P.E. Interactions between visual working memory and selective attention. *Psychol. Sci.* **2000**, *11*, 467–473. [CrossRef] [PubMed]

33. Lean, G.; (Ken) Clements, M.A. Spatial ability, visual imagery, and mathematical performance. *Educ. Stud. Math.* **1981**, *12*, 267–299. [CrossRef]

34. Mewborn, C.; Terry, D.; Lindbergh, C.; Renzi-Hammond, L.; Hammond, B.; Miller, L. Aging and Dementia-2Retinal and Serum Lutein and Zeaxanthin: Relation to white Matter Integrity in Younger and Older Adults. *Arch. Clin. Neuropsychol.* **2016**, *31*, 573. [CrossRef]

35. Renzi, L.M.; Hammond, B.R. The relation between the macular carotenoids, lutein and zeaxanthin, and temporal vision. *Ophthalmic Physiol. Opt.* **2010**, *30*, 351–357. [CrossRef] [PubMed]

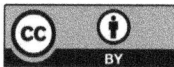

© 2017 by the authors. Licensee MDPI, Basel, Switzerland. This article is an open access article distributed under the terms and conditions of the Creative Commons Attribution (CC BY) license (http://creativecommons.org/licenses/by/4.0/).

nutrients

MDPI

Article

The Macular Carotenoids are Associated with Cognitive Function in Preadolescent Children

Sarah E. Saint [1,2,*], Lisa M. Renzi-Hammond [1,2], Naiman A. Khan [3], Charles H. Hillman [4], Janet E. Frick [1] and Billy R. Hammond Jr. [1]

[1] Department of Psychology, The University of Georgia, Athens, GA 30602, USA; lrenzi@uga.edu (L.M.R.-H.); jfrick@uga.edu (J.E.F.); bhammond@uga.edu (B.R.H.J.)

[2] Institute of Gerontology, Department of Health Promotion and Behavior, College of Public Health, The University of Georgia, Athens, GA 30602, USA

[3] The University of Illinois at Urbana-Champaign, Department of Kinesiology and Community Health, Champaign, IL 61820, USA; nakhan2@illinois.edu

[4] Departments of Psychology and Physical Therapy, Movement & Rehabilitation Sciences, Northeastern University, Boston, MA 02115, USA; c.hillman@northeastern.edu

* Correspondence: saints@uga.edu; Tel.: +1-706-542-4337

Received: 6 December 2017; Accepted: 6 February 2018; Published: 10 February 2018

Abstract: The macular carotenoids lutein (L) and zeaxanthin (Z) are obtained via diet and accumulate in the central retina where they are referred to as macular pigment. The density of this biomarker (macular pigment optical density; MPOD) has been positively correlated with cognitive functioning via measures of global cognition, processing speed, and visual-spatial abilities, among others. Although improvements in cognitive function have been found in adults, much less is known about how L and Z intake may support or improve cognitive functioning during periods of rapid developmental change, such as childhood and pre-adolescence. This study examined the relationship between MPOD and cognitive functioning in 51 7–13-year-old children (51% female). MPOD was measured using heterochromatic flicker photometry (HFP) optimized for this age group. Cognitive function was assessed using the Woodcock-Johnson III (composite standard scores were obtained for Brief Intellectual Ability, Verbal Ability, Cognitive Efficiency, Processing Speed, and Executive Processes). In this sample, MPOD was significantly related to Executive Processes, $r(47) = 0.288$, $p < 0.05$, and Brief Intellectual Ability, $r(47) = 0.268$, $p < 0.05$. The relationship to Cognitive Efficiency was positive and trending but not significant, $r(49) = 0.206$, $p = 0.074$. In general, these data are consistent with those of adults showing a link between higher carotenoid status and improved cognitive functioning.

Keywords: macular pigment; lutein; cognition; children

1. Introduction

The carotenoids lutein (L) and zeaxanthin (Z) are found in highest concentrations in dark green leafy vegetables (e.g., kale and spinach) and, when present in the diet, accumulate in the central retina where they are referred to collectively as macular pigment. In the retina, these pigments (along with their isomer, meso-zeaxanthin) serve as intraocular light filters, absorbing short-wavelength "blue" light (peak absorption at 460 nm) before it can reach the macula and damage the photoreceptors responsible for central vision. L and Z are also potent antioxidants and anti-inflammatory agents that help to protect the central nervous system from oxidative and inflammatory stress [1,2]. The brain and eye are particularly susceptible to free radical damage because they both have very high concentrations of polyunsaturated fatty acids and a high metabolic load.

Like many naturally derived compounds, the effects of L and Z on human biology are pleiotropic [3]; emerging research, for instance, has demonstrated a relationship between the macular carotenoids and cognitive performance in adults (see [4] for a review). There is reason to believe that these molecules may also be important for cognitive development in early life, but the relationship between L and Z status, measured directly in the central nervous system, and cognitive performance has only recently been examined in children [5–7].

An effect of L and Z on the developing retina/brain is biologically feasible [8]. L is the predominant carotenoid in the developing fetal and infant brain, despite relatively low dietary intake, and makes up 59% of the carotenoids in the infant brain [9] compared to 34% in geriatric adults [10]. It has been suggested that such high concentrations of L in the developing brain are an indication that it may be necessary during periods of rapid neural development [8,11,12]. Development is a time characterized by increased vulnerability to oxidative and inflammatory stress [13] and children tend to have significantly lower intake of L and Z compared to adults [14]. When studied in model cell cultures, carotenoids have been shown to promote the formation of gap junctions between cells [15]. Promoting gap junction communication would allow neurons to communicate laterally via direct ion exchange. This may improve cell-to-cell communication and could lead to faster and more efficient processing within the visual system, as well as throughout the central nervous system (i.e., the neural efficiency hypothesis [16,17]). Evidence showing that L and Z supplementation increases visual processing speed [18,19] is consistent with this possibility.

A number of studies have shown that higher L and Z predict better cognitive outcomes [5,7,20–23]. For example, low macular pigment optical density (MPOD) in a sample of older adults was associated with significantly lower performance on global measures of cognitive functioning (mini-mental status exam (MMSE) and Montreal Cognitive Assessment (MoCA)), as well as prospective memory and processing speed tasks [21]. MPOD has also been associated with attention and cognitive flexibility (as assessed by task switching), as well as visual memory and learning (paired associate learning task) in both healthy adults and those with retinal disease [24]. Older adults with higher MPOD exhibited less brain activation to complete a verbal learning task in a recent fMRI study [25].

Intervention trials with L and Z have yielded similar findings. For example, healthy older women who were supplemented with L, docosahexaeonic acid (DHA, an omega-3 fatty acid), or a combination of L and DHA showed improved verbal fluency in all three groups, as well as improvements in performance on several delayed recall memory tests in the L + DHA group [20]. A recent placebo-controlled trial involving older adults found that supplementation with L and Z improved performance on measures of complex attention and executive functions (i.e., cognitive flexibility) [23].

Similar observations have been made even in the very young. For example, infant recognition memory, tested using an event-related potential (ERP) oddball paradigm, has been positively associated with the amount of L and choline in mother's breastmilk [26]. MPOD, measured in preadolescent children, has been shown to associate positively with educational achievement (math and written comprehension) [5], aspects of relational memory on a spatial reconstruction task [7], as well as cognitive control performance and ERP outcomes on an attentional inhibition task [6].

These past studies have shown that MPOD can predict academic performance (math and written comprehension) and lab-based cognitive outcomes in preadolescent children. Whether MPOD can also predict outcomes on standardized tests of cognition, as it has been shown to do in adults [27], has yet to be determined. The present study tests the hypothesis that MPOD will positively correlate with performance on standardized cognitive assessments of global intelligence, verbal ability, cognitive efficiency, processing speed, and executive processes using the standardized Woodcock Johnson III Tests of Cognitive Abilities [28].

2. Materials and Methods

2.1. Participants

Fifty-four children (45.5% female) were recruited from the Athens, Georgia community. Data from three of these children were excluded from all analyses for the following reasons: (a) $n = 2$ participants had diagnoses that made testing (cognitive and/or MPOD) challenging (i.e., sensory processing disorder, ADHD), and (b) $n = 1$ participant was an outlier on the cognitive outcomes and complained of excessive fatigue (not characteristic of other subjects) during testing. The final sample consisted of 51 children (49% female). Children ranged in age from 7 to 13 and were largely white (non-Hispanic; 76.5%) and from well-educated families (90.2% of children had at least one parent with some level of post-secondary education). See Table 1 for complete demographic information. All participants had normal (or corrected-to-normal) vision while completing the tasks. Informed consent was obtained prior to participation from each participant's accompanying parent/guardian, in addition to the participant's assent, which was given verbally and/or in writing after an age-appropriate discussion of the study and what is meant by "voluntary participation". All study activities were carried out in accordance with the Declaration of Helsinki, and the study protocol was approved by the Ethics Committee of the University of Georgia (Study ID: 2013100730).

Table 1. Descriptive statistics for all participants included in analyses.

	N (%)
Age (years)	
7	16 (31.4)
8	5 (9.8)
9	9 (17.6)
10	6 (11.8)
11	8 (15.7)
12	6 (11.8)
13	1 (2.0)
Sex	
Male	26 (51.0)
Female	25 (49.0)
Race	
White (Non-Hispanic)	39 (76.5)
Hispanic	1 (2.0)
>1 Race Listed	11 (21.6)
Parent Highest Education	
High School or less	3 (5.9)
College Degree (AS, BS, BA)	18 (35.3)
Graduate Degree	28 (54.9)

2.2. Measures

2.2.1. Macular Pigment Optical Density (MPOD)

MPOD was measured using customized heterochromatic flicker photometry (HFP) via a Macular Densitometer™ (Macular Metrics Corporation, Rehoboth, MA, USA) as described in [29]. Measurement of MPOD in children using HFP has been demonstrated to be possible with a moderate degree of reliability (Cronbach's $\alpha = 0.72$) [30]. The standard one-degree and 460 nm test stimulus was used and the procedure largely followed that described in [30]. One difference from [30] in the present study is that testing was confined to only two experimenters who had extensive experience working with children, and the method of adjustment was used.

2.2.2. Cognitive Testing

Selected tests from the Woodcock-Johnson III (WJ-III) Tests of Cognitive Abilities [28] were used to assess children's cognitive functioning. The WJ-III is a norm-referenced set of tests designed to measure intellectual abilities in 2- to 90+-year-olds. The WJ-III was designed using the Cattell-Horn-Carroll Theory of Cognitive Abilities and has been standardized on over 8000 individuals who are representative of the demographics and communities of the general United States population [31]. All subtests of interest for this study have median reliability scores of 0.8 or higher, with the exception of the Planning subtest (median reliability = 0.75) [31]. All Cognitive Performance Composite scores of interest have median reliability scores of 0.9 or higher [31].

Participants completed the following WJ-III standard battery subtests: Verbal Comprehension, Concept Formation, Visual Matching 2, Numbers Reversed, Decision Speed, Planning, and Pair Cancellation. These subtests were chosen so that the following cognitive performance cluster scores could be calculated: Brief Intellectual Ability (BIA), Verbal Ability, Cognitive Efficiency, Processing Speed, and Executive Processes. Time constraints prevented the administration of the entire WJ-III standard battery, therefore these cluster scores were selected as being most likely to be related to levels of L and Z in the CNS based on previous work with adults, children, and infants [20–23,26].

One trained experimenter was responsible for testing all of the participants to reduce potential inter-rater reliability confounds. Participants were allowed to take breaks between subtests, and the order in which subtests were completed was altered as needed to maintain attention. For example, the Concept Formation subtest is particularly challenging, and participants frequently feel cognitively fatigued by the time that test is administered. On occasion, that subtest was moved to a later point in the testing session to allow participants to recover their attention during the more hands-on tasks (e.g., Visual Matching 2, Decision Speed, Planning, and Pair Cancellation) before attempting the more challenging Concept Formation task. Completion of these WJ-III subtests took 90 min to two hours. The decision to alter the order of subtest administration was made during the testing session based on experimenter judgment of the participant's level of fatigue.

2.3. Statistical Analyses

Statistical analyses were performed using SPSS version 24 (IBM, Armonk, NY, USA) and $\alpha = 0.05$ was used as the cutoff value for statistical significance. Bivariate correlations were calculated between MPOD and all cognitive variables, and one-tailed test values are reported (unless otherwise specified) given the directional nature of all a priori hypotheses (i.e., higher MPOD is associated with higher cognitive functioning). Partial correlations were calculated when necessary to control for sex or age differences. The distributional shapes of the MPOD and cognitive composite score variables were examined and found to meet the assumption of normality ($S\text{-}W \geq 0.967$, $df = 49$, $p \geq 0.181$ for all variables).

3. Results

The standard scores for the WJ-III Brief Intellectual Ability, Processing Speed, Cognitive Efficiency, and Executive Processes composite measures were used to assess specific components of cognitive functioning to control for age differences among participants. Four of the children tested were born prematurely (<37 weeks gestation). Given that prematurity has been linked to deficits in processing speed and academic achievement into adolescence [32,33], independent-samples t-tests were conducted to determine whether any differences in cognitive or visual performance existed based on prematurity. No significant differences were found for either measure (visual or cognitive), therefore these children were kept in the data set. Sex differences in WJ-III performance were detected for the Processing Speed composite score and Visual-Auditory Learning subtest; female participants demonstrated higher performance on both measures, $t(49) = -2.795$, $p = 0.007$ and $t(49) = -2.119$, $p = 0.039$ (two-tailed), respectively. Sex differences were not detected for MPOD or any other cognitive variables.

Two participants (7- and 10-years-old) were unwilling to complete the Concept Formation subtest of the WJ-III, which is required to calculate the BIA and Executive Processes composite scores, resulting in missing data for those variables. Additionally, one 7-year-old was unwilling to complete the Spatial Relations subtest. Final sample size and descriptive statistics for all measures can be found in Table 2.

MPOD was significantly related to global intelligence (Brief Intellectual Ability; BIA) and Executive Processes composite scores (age-normed; see Table 3 and Figure 1). In addition, the relationship between MPOD and Cognitive Efficiency approached significance, $r(49) = 0.206$, $p = 0.074$ (one-tailed). The Verbal Learning and Processing Speed measures were not significantly related to MPOD (see Table 3; both $ps > 0.10$, one-tailed).

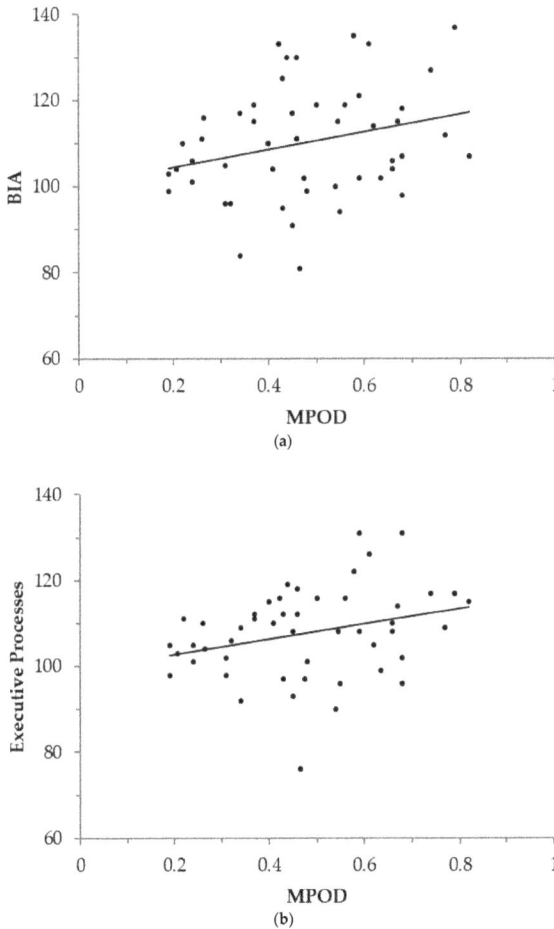

Figure 1. The relationship between macular pigment optical density (MPOD) and the following WJ-III Cognitive Composite scores: (**a**) Brief Intellectual Ability (BIA), regression line constant = 100.295, $\beta = 20.523$, $R^2(47) = 0.072$, and (**b**) Executive Processes, regression line constant = 99.234, $\beta = 17.705$, $R^2(47) = 0.083$. Standard scores were used for all cognitive variables to control for age. Note: Regression equations were calculated with MPOD predicting cognitive performance, though it should be noted that the correlational design of the present study does not allow for causal interpretations.

Exploratory analyses were performed using MPOD and two WJ-III subtests that were not included in the calculation of the cluster scores reported above. Performance on the Spatial Relations subtest (a measure of visual-spatial thinking abilities) was positively related to MPOD, $r(48) = 0.299$, $p = 0.035$ (two-tailed; see Figure 2), while the partial correlation controlling for sex between MPOD and performance on the Visual-Auditory Learning subtest (a measure of paired-associate learning) did not reach significance, $r(48) = 0.236$, $p = 0.099$ (two-tailed; see Table 4).

Table 2. Descriptive statistics for all measures.

	Mean	SD	Range	N
MPOD	0.476	0.167	0.190–0.820	51
Cognitive Measures (All Standard Scores)				
WJ-III Composite Scores				
Brief Intellectual Ability (BIA)	110.10	13.012	81–137	49
Verbal Ability	112.41	12.420	89–144	51
Cognitive Efficiency	104.02	15.909	65–132	51
Processing Speed	100.10	17.258	75–151	51
Executive Processes	107.69	10.453	76–131	49
Select WJ-III Subtests				
Visual-Auditory Learning	100.84	13.249	75–132	51
Spatial Relations	108.48	13.526	72–132	50

Note: MPOD = Macular Pigment Optical Density. SD: standard deviation.

Table 3. Correlations among MPOD and WJ-III cognitive cluster scores. All correlations are bivariate with the exception of Processing Speed, which was calculated as a partial correlation controlling for sex, given that sex differences were evident in the Processing Speed variable.

	BIA	Verbal Ability	Cognitive Efficiency	Processing Speed	Executive Processes
MPOD	0.268 * (N = 49)	0.159 (N = 51)	0.206 † (N = 51)	0.099 (N = 51)	0.288 * (N = 49)

* $p < 0.05$, † $p \leq 0.10$ (one-tailed). Note: MPOD = Macular Pigment Optical Density. BIA = Brief Intellectual Ability. The number of subjects who completed each set of measures is reported in parentheses below each correlation.

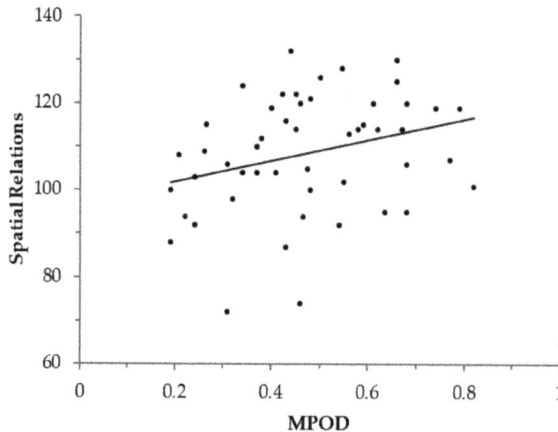

Figure 2. The relationship between macular pigment optical density (MPOD) and the WJ-III Spatial Relations subtest, regression line constant = 97.073, $\beta = 24.081$, $R^2(48) = 0.090$. Standard scores were used for Spatial Relations variable to control for age. Note: Regression equation was calculated with MPOD predicting cognitive performance, though it should be noted that the correlational design of the present study does not allow for causal interpretations.

Table 4. Correlations among MPOD and two WJ-III cognitive subtests of interest. The correlation between MPOD and Visual-Auditory Learning was calculated as a partial correlation controlling for sex, given that sex differences were evident in that cognitive subtest.

	Spatial Relations	Visual-Auditory Learning
MPOD	0.299 * (N = 50)	0.236 † (N = 51)

* $p < 0.05$, † $p \leq 0.10$ (two-tailed). Note: MPOD = Macular Pigment Optical Density. The number of subjects who completed each set of measures is reported in parentheses below each correlation.

4. Discussion

The present study tested whether MPOD, a marker of macular pigments L and Z concentration in the retina, related to standardized measures of cognitive functioning in pre-adolescent children. MPOD correlates highly with levels of lutein in the brain [34] and is therefore considered a reliable biomarker of overall central nervous system carotenoid status. Our findings further demonstrate that the ability to measure these carotenoids directly within neural tissue is a unique and powerful approach to assess the role these phytochemicals play in that very tissue: MPOD was positively related to global intelligence (BIA), executive functioning, and visuo-spatial thinking abilities in this sample of preadolescent children. In addition, the relationship between MPOD and cognitive efficiency approached significance.

These cognitive processes are founded in networks involving the frontal and parietal cortices, with input from the occipital cortex (as well as other regions), and the frontal and occipital cortices are brain regions that contain particularly high concentrations of L and Z, when they are present in diet [34]. Our results are in general agreement with data collected from adult and aging populations, as well as recent studies of other samples of preadolescent children [5–7,20–23]. Higher MPOD has been associated with higher cognitive performance in a number of areas. For example, MPOD relates to measures of global cognitive functioning and executive functioning in older adults [21,23]. These types of cognitive effects have also been manifest when using neuroimaging tools. For example, studies using fMRI have shown that higher MPOD is related to greater efficiency in the form of reduced brain activation during task execution in adults [25], and EEG work has demonstrated better cognitive control in both young children and adults [6,22].

Children's scores on the WJ-III Processing Speed composite measure were not related to MPOD in the present study. The tests that make up the WJ-III Processing Speed Composite score require children to circle items on a page (given various rules, such as "circle the two items in each row that are most alike" or "circle the two numbers in each row that are the same") as fast as they can until they reach the end or three minutes has passed. Despite the "speed" designation, this test is unlike other measures of processing speed, such as critical flicker fusion frequency (CFF), that are significantly related to MPOD in young adults [16–18]. Tasks such as CFF are atomistic in nature. They are limited by the transmission speed of neurons within the visual cortex and do not reflect the additional processing necessary for decision-making and understanding relationships between items in categories, which are largely frontal lobe phenomena [35].

These results highlight the importance of diet in supporting cognitive health in preadolescent children. It is likely that the participants tested in our study (similar to those tested in [30]) may reflect less deficiency than is often seen in the average American diet given the sample was collected in a large public university-based community (our average MPOD was relatively high). The latest National Health and Nutrition Examination Survey (NHANES) fruit and vegetable intake report reveals that dark green vegetables were consumed by only 10.7% of US children between the ages of 6–11 on a given day in 2009–2010 [36]. This dietary behavior is reflected in relatively low average intake of L and Z (about three times lower than adults) [14] and suggest that this dietary behavior may be worsening over time. Children under the age of 12 decreased their yearly vegetable intake between 2009 and 2015 by 12 servings per capita [37]. The present study was not designed to establish a causal relationship between MPOD (or L and Z intake) and cognition, but given the cross-sectional relationships between L and Z with cognitive outcomes in children, future studies should attempt to do so. This could be done by increasing L and Z intake in children via supplementation or dietary interventions to determine whether children also exhibit the same positive benefits that adult supplementation studies have demonstrated [18,20,23].

Acknowledgments: The authors would like to thank Lloyd Stephen Miller for his feedback and suggestions. Funding Source: Research support was provided by Abbott Nutrition through the Center for Nutrition, Learning, and Memory (CNLM) at the University of Illinois, Urbana-Champaign.

Author Contributions: L.M.R.-H., B.R.H.J., N.A.K. and C.H.H. conceived and designed the experiments; S.E.S. and L.M.R.-H. performed the experiments; S.E.S. analyzed the data; S.E.S., B.R.H.J., L.M.R.-H., C.H.H., N.A.K. and J.E.F. wrote the paper.

Conflicts of Interest: The authors declare no conflict of interest. The founding sponsors had no role in the design of the study; in the collection, analyses, or interpretation of data; in the writing of the manuscript, and in the decision to publish the results.

References

1. Stahl, W.; Sies, H. Antioxidant activity of carotenoids. *Mol. Asp. Med.* **2003**, *24*, 345–351. [CrossRef]
2. Ozawa, Y.; Sasaki, M.; Takahashi, N.; Kamoshita, M.; Miyake, S.; Tsubota, K. Neuroprotective Effects of Lutein in the Retina. *Curr. Pharm. Des.* **2012**, *18*, 51–56. [CrossRef] [PubMed]
3. Hammond, B. Lutein's Influence on Neural Processing Speed. In Proceedings of the 114th Abbott Nutrition Research Conference, Cognition and nutrition, Columbus, OH, USA, 8–9 April 2013; pp. 1–6.
4. Jia, Y.P.; Sun, L.; Yu, H.S.; Liang, L.P.; Li, W.; Ding, H.; Song, X.B.; Zhang, L.J. The pharmacological effects of lutein and zeaxanthin on visual disorders and cognition diseases. *Molecules* **2017**, *22*, 610. [CrossRef] [PubMed]
5. Barnett, S.M.; Khan, N.A.; Walk, A.M.; Raine, L.B.; Moulton, C.; Cohen, N.J.; Kramer, A.F.; Hammond, B.R.; Renzi-Hammond, L.; Hillman, C.H. Macular pigment optical density is positively associated with academic performance among preadolescent children. *Nutr. Neurosci.* **2017**, *8305*, 1–9. [CrossRef] [PubMed]
6. Walk, A.M.; Khan, N.A.; Barnett, S.M.; Raine, L.B.; Kramer, A.F.; Cohen, N.J.; Moulton, C.J.; Renzi-Hammond, L.M.; Hammond, B.R.; Hillman, C.H. From neuro-pigments to neural efficiency: The relationship between retinal carotenoids and behavioral and neuroelectric indices of cognitive control in childhood. *Int. J. Psychophysiol.* **2017**, *118*, 1–8. [CrossRef] [PubMed]
7. Hassevoort, K.M.; Khazoum, S.E.; Walker, J.A.; Barnett, S.M.; Raine, L.B.; Hammond, B.R.; Renzi-Hammond, L.M.; Kramer, A.F.; Khan, N.A.; Hillman, C.H.; et al. Macular Carotenoids, Aerobic Fitness, and Central Adiposity Are Associated Differentially with Hippocampal-Dependent Relational Memory in Preadolescent Children. *J. Pediatr.* **2017**, *183*, 108–114. [CrossRef] [PubMed]
8. Hammond, B.R. The Dietary Carotenoids Lutein and Zeaxanthin in Pre-and-Postnatal Development. *Funct. Food Rev.* **2012**, *4*, 130–137. [CrossRef]
9. Vishwanathan, R.; Kuchan, M.J.; Sen, S.; Johnson, E.J. Lutein and preterm infants with decreased concentrations of brain carotenoids. *J. Pediatr. Gastroenterol. Nutr.* **2014**, *59*, 659–665. [CrossRef] [PubMed]
10. Johnson, E.J.; Vishwanathan, R.; Johnson, M.A.; Hausman, D.B.; Davey, A.; Scott, T.M.; Green, R.C.; Miller, L.S.; Gearing, M.; Woodard, J.; et al. Relationship between serum and brain carotenoids, α-tocopherol, and retinol concentrations and cognitive performance in the oldest old from the Georgia centenarian study. *J. Aging Res.* **2013**, *2013*, 951786. [CrossRef] [PubMed]
11. Hammond, B.R. Possible role for dietary lutein and zeaxanthin in visual development. *Nutr. Rev.* **2008**, *66*, 695–702. [CrossRef] [PubMed]
12. Johnson, E.J. Role of lutein and zeaxanthin in visual and cognitive function throughout the lifespan. *Nutr. Rev.* **2014**, *72*, 605–612. [CrossRef] [PubMed]
13. Holt, E.M.; Steffen, L.M.; Moran, A.; Basu, S.; Steinberger, J.; Ross, J.A.; Hong, C.P.; Sinaiko, A.R. Fruit and Vegetable Consumption and Its Relation to Markers of Inflammation and Oxidative Stress in Adolescents. *J. Am. Diet. Assoc.* **2009**, *109*, 414–421. [CrossRef] [PubMed]
14. Johnson, E.J.; Maras, J.E.; Rasmussen, H.M.; Tucker, K.L. Intake of Lutein and Zeaxanthin Differ with Age, Sex, and Ethnicity. *J. Am. Diet. Assoc.* **2010**, *110*, 1357–1362. [CrossRef] [PubMed]

15. Stahl, W.; Sies, H. Effects of carotenoids and retinoids on gap junctional communication. *BioFactors* **2001**, *15*, 95–98. [CrossRef] [PubMed]

16. Hammond, B.R.; Wooten, B.R. CFF thresholds: Relation to macular pigment optical density. *Ophthalmic Physiol. Opt.* **2005**, *25*, 315–319. [CrossRef] [PubMed]

17. Renzi, L.M.; Hammond, B.R. The relation between the macular carotenoids, lutein and zeaxanthin, and temporal vision. *Ophthalmic Physiol. Opt.* **2010**, *30*, 351–357. [CrossRef] [PubMed]

18. Bovier, E.R.; Renzi, L.M.; Hammond, B.R. A double-blind, placebo-controlled study on the effects of lutein and zeaxanthin on neural processing speed and efficiency. *PLoS ONE* **2014**, *9*, e108178. [CrossRef] [PubMed]

19. Bovier, E.R.; Hammond, B.R. A randomized placebo-controlled study on the effects of lutein and zeaxanthin on visual processing speed in young healthy subjects. *Arch. Biochem. Biophys.* **2015**, *572*, 54–57. [CrossRef] [PubMed]

20. Johnson, E.; McDonald, K.; Caldarella, S.; Chung, H.-Y.; Troen, A.; Snodderly, D. Cognitive findings of an exploratory trial of docosahexaenoic acid and lutein supplementation in older women. *Nutr. Neurosci.* **2008**, *11*, 75–83. [CrossRef] [PubMed]

21. Feeney, J.; Finucane, C.; Savva, G.M.; Cronin, H.; Beatty, S.; Nolan, J.M.; Kenny, R.A. Low macular pigment optical density is associated with lower cognitive performance in a large, population-based sample of older adults. *Neurobiol. Aging* **2013**, *34*, 2449–2456. [CrossRef] [PubMed]

22. Walk, A.M.; Edwards, C.G.; Baumgartner, N.W.; Curran, M.R.; Covello, A.R.; Reeser, G.E.; Hammond, B.R.; Renzi, L.M.; Khan, N.A. The Role of Retinal Carotenoids and Age on Neuroelectric Indices of Attentional Control among early to middle-aged adults. *Front. Aging Neurosci.* **2017**, *9*, 1–13. [CrossRef] [PubMed]

23. Hammond, B.R.; Stephen Miller, L.; Bello, M.O.; Lindbergh, C.A.; Mewborn, C.; Renzi-Hammond, L.M. Effects of lutein/zeaxanthin supplementation on the cognitive function of community dwelling older adults: A randomized, double-masked, placebo-controlled trial. *Front. Aging Neurosci.* **2017**, *9*, 1–9. [CrossRef] [PubMed]

24. Kelly, D.; Coen, R.F.; Akuffo, K.O.; Beatty, S.; Dennison, J.; Moran, R.; Stack, J.; Howard, A.N.; Mulcahy, R.; Nolan, J.M. Cognitive function and its relationship with macular pigment optical density and serum concentrations of its constituent carotenoids. *J. Alzheimer's Dis.* **2015**, *48*, 261–277. [CrossRef] [PubMed]

25. Lindbergh, C.A.; Mewborn, C.M.; Hammond, B.R.; Renzi-Hammond, L.M.; Curran-Celentano, J.M.; Miller, L.S. Relationship of lutein and zeaxanthin levels to neurocognitive functioning: An fMRI study of older adults. *J. Int. Neuropsychol. Soc.* **2016**, *22*, 1–12. [CrossRef] [PubMed]

26. Cheatham, C.L.; Sheppard, K.W. Synergistic effects of human milk nutrients in the support of infant recognition memory: An observational study. *Nutrients* **2015**, *7*, 9079–9095. [CrossRef] [PubMed]

27. Renzi, L.M.; Dengler, M.J.; Puente, A.; Miller, L.S.; Hammond, B.R. Relationships between macular pigment optical density and cognitive function in unimpaired and mildly cognitively impaired older adults. *Neurobiol. Aging* **2014**, *35*, 1695–1699. [CrossRef] [PubMed]

28. Woodcock, R.W.; McGrew, K.S.; Mather, N. *Woodcock-Johnson III Tests of Cognitive Abilities*; Riverside: Rolling Meadows, IL, USA, 2001.

29. Wooten, B.R.; Hammond, B.R.; Land, R.I.; Snodderly, D.M. A practical method for measuring macular pigment optical density. *Investig. Ophthalmol. Vis. Sci.* **1999**, *40*, 2481–2489.

30. McCorkle, S.; Raine, L.; Hammond, B.; Renzi-Hammond, L.; Hillman, C.; Khan, N. Reliability of heterochromatic flicker photometry in measuring macular pigment optical density among preadolescent children. *Foods* **2015**, *4*, 594–604. [CrossRef] [PubMed]

31. Mather, N.; Woodcock, R.W. *Examiner's Manual: Woodcock-Johnson III Tests of Cognitive Abilities*; Riverside: Rolling Meadows, IL, USA, 2001.

32. Rose, S.; Feldman, J.; Jankowski, J.; Van Rossem, R. Basic information processing abilities at 11years account for deficits in IQ associated with preterm birth. *Intelligence* **2011**, *39*, 198–209. [CrossRef] [PubMed]

33. Rose, S.; Feldman, J.; Jankowski, J. Implications of infant cognition for executive functions at age 11. *Psychol. Sci.* **2012**, *23*, 1345–1355. [CrossRef] [PubMed]

34. Vishwanathan, R.; Neuringer, M.; Snodderly, D.M.; Schalch, W.; Johnson, E.J. Macular lutein and zeaxanthin are related to brain lutein and zeaxanthin in primates. *Nutr. Neurosci.* **2013**, *16*, 21–29. [CrossRef] [PubMed]

35. Mishkin, M.; Weiskrantz, L. Effects of cortical lesions in monkeys on critical flicker frequency. *J. Comp. Physiol. Psychol.* **1959**, *52*, 660. [CrossRef] [PubMed]

36. Nielsen, S.J.; Rossen, L.M.; Harris, D.M.; Ogden, C.L. *Fruit and Vegetable Consumption of U.S. Youth, 2009–2010*; U.S. Department of Health and Human Services, Centers for Disease Control and Prevention, National Center for Health Statistics: Hyattsville, MD, USA, 2014.
37. Produce for Better Health Foundation. State of the Plate, 2015 Study on America's Consumption of Fruit and Vegetables. 2015. Available online: http://www.pbhfoundation.org (accessed on 5 December 2017).

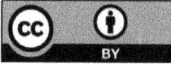

© 2018 by the authors. Licensee MDPI, Basel, Switzerland. This article is an open access article distributed under the terms and conditions of the Creative Commons Attribution (CC BY) license (http://creativecommons.org/licenses/by/4.0/).

nutrients

MDPI

Article

Lutein and Zeaxanthin Are Positively Associated with Visual–Spatial Functioning in Older Adults: An fMRI Study

Catherine M. Mewborn [1], Cutter A. Lindbergh [1], Talia L. Robinson [1], Marissa A. Gogniat [1], Douglas P. Terry [2], Kharine R. Jean [1], Billy Randy Hammond [1], Lisa M. Renzi-Hammond [1,3] and Lloyd Stephen Miller [1,*]

[1] Department of Psychology, The University of Georgia, Athens, GA 30602, USA; cmewborn@uga.edu (C.M.M.); cal@uga.edu (C.A.L.); talia.robinson25@uga.edu (T.L.R.); marissa.gogniat25@uga.edu (M.A.G.); kjean@uga.edu (K.R.J.); bhammond@uga.edu (B.R.H.); lrenzi@uga.edu (L.M.R.-H.)
[2] Department of Physical Medicine and Rehabilitation, Department of Psychiatry, Massachusetts General Hospital, Boston, MA 02114, USA; douglasterry1@gmail.com
[3] Institute of Gerontology, Department of Health Promotions and Behavior, College of Public Health, The University of Georgia, Athens, GA 30602, USA
* Correspondence: lsmiller@uga.edu; Tel.: +1-706-542-1173

Received: 8 March 2018; Accepted: 4 April 2018; Published: 7 April 2018

Abstract: Lutein (L) and zeaxanthin (Z) are two xanthophyll carotenoids that have antioxidant and anti-inflammatory properties. Previous work has demonstrated their importance for eye health and preventing diseases such as age-related macular degeneration. An emerging literature base has also demonstrated the importance of L and Z in cognition, neural structure, and neural efficiency. The present study aimed to better understand the mechanisms by which L and Z relate to cognition, in particular, visual–spatial processing and decision-making in older adults. We hypothesized that markers of higher levels of L and Z would be associated with better neural efficiency during a visual–spatial processing task. L and Z were assessed via standard measurement of blood serum and retinal concentrations. Visual–spatial processing and decision-making were assessed via a judgment of line orientation task (JLO) completed during a functional magnetic resonance imaging (fMRI) scan. The results demonstrated that individuals with higher concentrations of L and Z showed a decreased blood-oxygen-level dependent (BOLD) signal during task performance (i.e., "neural efficiency") in key areas associated with visual–spatial perception, processing, decision-making, and motor coordination, including the lateral occipital cortex, occipital pole, superior and middle temporal gyri, superior parietal lobule, superior and middle frontal gyri, and pre- and post-central gyri. To our knowledge, this is the first investigation of the relationship of L and Z to visual–spatial processing at a neural level using in vivo methodology. Our findings suggest that L and Z may impact brain health and cognition in older adults by enhancing neurobiological efficiency in a variety of regions that support visual perception and decision-making.

Keywords: xanthophylls; visual-spatial reasoning; fMRI; older adults; cognition

1. Introduction

Previous research has increasingly demonstrated the importance of diet and nutritional factors in brain health, especially in older adults [1]. Lutein (L) and zeaxanthin (Z) are two xanthophyll carotenoids that are acquired predominantly through the consumption of green leafy vegetables and brightly colored fruit and have previously been shown to positively relate to neurocognitive functioning [2]. Relative to other carotenoids present in human sera, L and Z preferentially cross the blood–brain barrier and accumulate in brain tissue, where they account for 66–77% of the total carotenoid concentration [3]. L and Z have been found to accumulate throughout diffuse regions of the brain, including the frontal, temporal, and occipital cortices, as well as the cerebellum and pons [3–5].

Historically, L and Z have been studied in relation to eye health, revealing their protective roles against age-related macular degeneration and the development of other optical diseases [6,7]. Previous literature has also demonstrated a positive relationship between intake of L and Z and better performance on a range of cognitive tasks, including executive functioning, learning and memory, verbal fluency, and processing speed [8–12]. Of particular relevance to this study, L and Z have been shown to positively relate to many aspects of visual–spatial functioning, including perceptual abilities, perceptual speed, and visual–spatial constructional skills [9,11]. Although this body of literature is still developing, there is evidence to suggest that L and Z may be two dietary factors that are important for a range of cognitive outcomes.

L and Z are primarily measured via concentrations in serum and the retina. Serum levels of L and Z are strongly related to recent dietary intake of foods rich in these nutrients [13]. In the retina, L and Z preferentially accumulate in the macula, where their concentrations can be assessed by measuring macular pigment optical density (MPOD), a validated measure of L and Z concentrations [14]. Because of the close relationship between the retina and the rest of the central nervous system, MPOD is considered a proxy for neural L and Z concentrations [5]. Although serum and retinal concentrations of L and Z are positively correlated, they are dissociable measures that may represent distinct aspects of dietary health [13,15,16]. For example, serum concentrations of L and Z are more variable than MPOD concentrations [17]. Additionally, after supplementation of L and Z, serum concentrations more quickly return to baseline levels whereas MPOD changes can last for several months [13]. Thus, serum concentrations of L and Z may more closely reflect acute dietary factors, whereas MPOD may reflect more stable L and Z levels that are acquired over a longer period of time.

Previous studies have demonstrated diffuse accumulation of L and Z in human brain tissue postmortem and have shown a positive relationship between concentrations of L and Z and performance on a wide range of cognitive tasks [2–4,8–12,18]. However, there is a lack of research investigating underlying neural mechanisms in vivo. To date, limited data exist that have examined the relationship between L and Z and neural structure and function using neuroimaging methodology. Our laboratory has conducted several investigations to address this gap in the literature using a sample of older adults enrolled in a nutrition intervention study. First, Lindbergh and colleagues (2017) assessed the cross-sectional relationship between serum and retinal concentrations of L and Z and brain activation during a verbal learning and memory fMRI task in our older adult sample [19]. The results indicated that greater L and Z levels were correlated with neural efficiency, as indicated by a decreased BOLD signal during task performance in several key brain regions for verbal learning and memory, including the central and parietal operculum, inferior frontal gyrus, supramarginal gyrus, planum polare, frontal and middle temporal gyrus, superior parietal lobule, pre- and post-central gyri, bilateral occipital cortex, and the cerebellum [19]. Another analysis from our laboratory, which used diffusion tensor imaging (DTI) in older adults, demonstrated that L and Z concentrations were positively correlated with measures of pre-intervention white matter integrity in major white matter tracts vulnerable to age-related decline, including the uncinate fasciculus and the cingulum [20]. Finally, in a pre-post intervention analysis of our sample, Lindbergh and colleagues (2018) found that L and Z supplementation increased cerebral perfusion and intensified neural responses in common brain regions at risk of deterioration in older adults, suggesting a possible neuroprotective effect of an L and Z intervention [21]. Other studies have also found L and Z to be related with better neural structure and function using structural MRI and EEG imaging technology [22,23]. Together, these findings offer a potential explanation for the mechanisms by which L and Z influence cognition, namely by bolstering neural structure and enhancing neural efficiency during cognitive task performance.

The current study aimed to further explore the mechanisms by which L and Z are related to cognitive functioning using functional magnetic resonance imaging (fMRI) in older adults. Given the importance of L and Z for visual health, we focused on the relationship between L and Z and performance during visual–spatial reasoning.

Visual–spatial reasoning is a domain of cognitive function that involves an individual's ability to perceive and organize visual stimuli. It includes a variety of related abilities, such as mental rotation, visual construction, and spatial orientation. Declines in visual–spatial abilities are associated both with normal [24,25] and pathological cognitive aging [26,27]. Visual–spatial reasoning is often impaired in the early stages of neurological disorders like Parkinson's disease [28,29] and may be an indicator of disease progression in Alzheimer's disease [30,31]. Additionally, visual–spatial abilities are important for functional competence in older adulthood [25,32]. For example, declines in spatial reasoning and orientation, in addition to memory and attention deficits, are associated with greater fall risk in older adults [33].

The Benton Judgment of Line Orientation (JLO) test is a commonly used measure of visual–spatial abilities that focuses specifically on spatial orientation, spatial judgment, and spatial reasoning [34]. Performance in visual–spatial reasoning tasks like the JLO is largely attributed to activation of right hemispheric structures [35–38]. Further exploration of neuroanatomical correlates of similar spatial reasoning tasks have consistently demonstrated evidence for the involvement of the right hemisphere, specifically the right parietal, parietal–temporal, and parietal–occipital regions [34,39]. More recent studies employing fMRI have consistently identified the right parietal and occipitoparietal involvement in JLO performance and similar orientation tasks, specifically activation in the right superior parietal cortex, angular gyrus, posterior supramarginal gyrus, and middle occipital gyrus [40–42]. Whereas parietal and occipital regions have been most consistently associated with performance in spatial orientation tasks, other regions have also been found to be associated with performance in visual–spatial reasoning tasks based on task difficulty. For example, Kesler and colleagues (2004) found that activation increased in frontal and occipital regions, in addition to the parietal region, as task difficulty in the JLO increased [41].

The right hemisphere is most closely associated with performance in visual–spatial tasks; however, left hemispheric involvement is also seen, particularly in older adults [41,43]. Previous work suggests that older adults compensate for age-related neural declines by recruiting more diverse brain regions and showing increased bilateralized brain activity while performing cognitively demanding tasks compared to the more focal activation seen in younger adults [43–45]. Although there has been limited work analyzing compensatory recruitment specifically during visual–spatial orientation tasks, there is evidence for differential activation and diminished specificity in regions of the brain related to processes such as visual recognition in healthy older adults compared to healthy young adults [46]. Other studies have similarly found diminished neural specificity in visual recognition and visual memory areas of the brain with increasing age [47,48].

In the current study, fMRI methodology was used to cross-sectionally assess the relationship between serum and retinal (MPOD) concentrations of L and Z and brain activity during performance on an fMRI-adapted JLO task [34] in a sample of community-dwelling older adults. In line with theories of compensatory brain aging, we hypothesized that L and Z concentrations would be negatively related to neural activity in parietal–temporal–occipital areas, including the superior parietal cortex, angular gyrus, supramarginal gyrus, and middle occipital gyrus, which have shown consistent involvement in performance of visual–spatial tasks [40–42]. In other words, individuals with lower concentrations of L and Z were expected to show a greater task-related BOLD signal (i.e., "neural inefficiency") during JLO performance relative to individuals with higher concentrations. Generally, we hypothesized that activation would be right-lateralized, but could not rule out left hemispheric involvement [41,43]. Behaviorally, we hypothesized a positive relationship between L and Z concentrations and JLO task accuracy. Given that serum and retinal concentrations of L and Z are related, yet distinct, measures, we expected congruent, but not necessarily identical, relationships of these two measures with neural activation in the hypothesized regions.

2. Materials and Methods

2.1. Subjects

The sample included 51 community-dwelling older adults (see Table 1 for demographic details). Participants were recruited as part of a larger, randomized-controlled trial of L and Z supplementation via newspaper advertisements, flyers, and a database of individuals who previously had consented to being contacted for future research studies. Data for this study are drawn from the baseline visits and are pre-supplementation. Exclusion criteria included left-handedness, history of ocular disease, corrected visual acuity of worse than 20:40 (Snellen notation), age-related macular degeneration in either eye, gastric conditions with the potential to interfere with L and Z absorption (e.g., gastric ulcer, Crohn's disease, ulcerative colitis), contraindications for safe MRI data collection (e.g., metallic implants), or history of traumatic brain injury, dementia, or other neurological disease.

Data for this study were collected across three baseline visits, with an additional blood draw to collect serum data that was scheduled at a time convenient for participants. Prior to enrollment in the study, exclusion criteria were assessed via a telephone screening. Potentially eligible participants completed a physical examination to confirm good health and eligibility for continued participation. During visit one, full informed consent was obtained, demographic information and other variables pertinent to the larger study were collected, and cognitive status was screened for using the Clinical Dementia Rating Scale (CDR) [49]. Individuals were excluded from further participation if they showed evidence of mild to severe dementia, as indicated by a CDR total score of 1–3. During visit two, participants completed vision testing to collect MPOD measurements and other variables pertinent to the larger study. During visit three, participants completed MRI data collection.

Serum L and Z data were not available for 5 participants; thus, analyses using serum were conducted with a smaller sub-group of participants ($n = 46$). This sub-group did not differ significantly from the larger sample with regard to age, sex, education, mean MPOD, or mean performance on the JLO task.

Table 1. Descriptive characteristics of participants, task performance, and lutein/zeaxanthin concentrations.

Age (Years)	Sex (% Female)	Race (% Caucasian)	Education (Years)	JLO Task Accuracy (Max = 60) [1]	MPOD (o.d.)	Serum L & Z (μmol/L) [2]
71.75 ± 6.16	58.8	100.0	16.1 ± 3.15	52.53 ± 4.49	0.495 ± 0.177	0.321 ± 0.170

JLO = Judgement of Line Orientation. MPOD = macular pigment optical density. o.d. = optical density, the log ratio of transmitted light passing through the macula. [1] Data available for 40 participants. [2] Data available for 46 participants.

2.2. Ethics

Informed consent was obtained from all participants. The study protocol was approved by the Institutional Review Board and the tenets of the Declaration of Helsinki were adhered to at all times by study personnel.

2.3. Methods

2.3.1. Visual Acuity

Self-reported visual acuity was confirmed via Snellen acuity testing as delineated in Levenson and Kozarsky (1990) [50].

2.3.2. Judgment of Line Orientation (JLO) Task

Participants completed a JLO task conceptually based on the Benton JLO task [34] and adapted for the fMRI environment by the experimenters. The task was programmed using E-Prime (version 1.2, Psychology Software Tools, Inc., Pittsburgh, PA, USA) and presented through MRI compatible goggles

(Resonance Technology Inc., Northridge, CA, USA). Prior to beginning the MRI, all participants were given a visual acuity test using the goggles to determine whether they could see the task clearly and accurately. Corrective lenses ranging from −9.0 to +3.0 were available to assist participants with myopia or hyperopia in viewing the task through the MRI compatible goggles. Participants responded using Cedrus Lumina LU400 MRI compatible response pads (Cedrus, San Pedro, CA, USA). The task consisted of 10 blocks each of active baseline and JLO task blocks (see Figure 1). During the active baseline blocks, participants were asked to assess whether two horizontal lines were in the same horizontal plane. Participants were instructed to respond using their right index finger if the two lines were horizontally even, or their left index finger if the two lines were uneven (maximum score = 30). Even and uneven line stimuli were presented in a random order with replacement. During the JLO task blocks, participants were asked to judge whether an angle presented in the top half of the screen matched an angle that was highlighted in red from an array of angles below. Participants were instructed to respond using their right index finger if the two angles matched, or their left index finger if the two angles did not match (maximum score = 30). During the JLO task blocks, stimuli were presented in sequential order from a library of 144 images. During each active baseline and JLO task block, ten stimuli were presented for three seconds each. Participants were trained on the JLO task outside of the scanner for approximately 30 min to ensure understanding of the task and task response instructions.

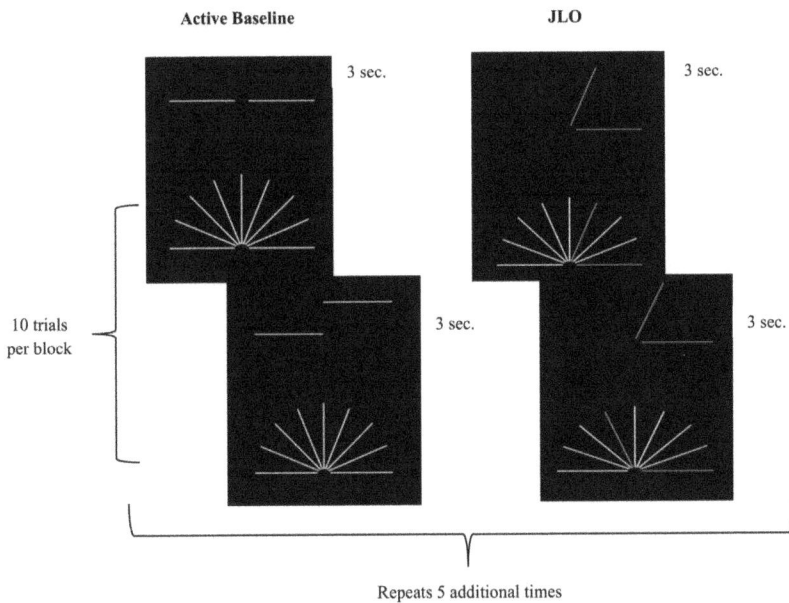

Figure 1. JLO task design. The figure provides a visual schematic of the judgement of line orientation (JLO) task. The two blocks (i.e., active baseline and JLO) were presented a total of six times, resulting in a total acquisition time of 6 min, 33 s. Ten stimuli were presented in each block in a random order with replacement for the active baseline and a sequential order from a library of 144 images for the JLO task.

2.3.3. Macular Pigment Optical Density (MPOD)

MPOD was assessed via customized heterochromatic flicker photometry (cHFP) using well-validated procedures [14,51,52]. Participants were shown a disc that was comprised of shortwave "blue light" (460 nanometer, nm) and midwave "green" light (570 nm). The two wavelengths of light are presented in square-wave, counter-phase orientation, which causes the stimulus disc to appear to "flicker." Participants adjust the intensity of the 460 nm light until it matches the luminance of the 570 nm light and the disc ceases to "flicker." Since the macular pigment strongly absorbs the 460 nm light, individuals with a denser macular pigment layer (thus a higher concentration of retinal L and Z) require more intense 460 nm to match the 570 nm light. This procedure was conducted in both the foveal and parafoveal regions of the retina and was customized for each individual participant based on their previously measured critical flicker fusion frequency (CFF). MPOD was calculated as the log intensity of the 460 nm light required to match the 570 nm light in the fovea versus the parafovea regions.

2.3.4. Serum Lutein and Zeaxanthin (Serum L & Z)

Full details of the serum L & Z analysis can be found elsewhere [19]. Briefly, 7 mL (mL) of blood was collected by a certified phlebotomist. Blood samples were placed on ice and centrifuged for 15 min after collection. Serum data were extracted using standard lipid extraction methods, and serum was frozen in 1 mL cryotubes at −80 °C until analysis. L and Z concentrations were analyzed using a Hewlett Packard/Agilent Technologies 1100 series high performance liquid chromatography (HPLC) system with a photodiode array detector (Agilent Technologies, Palo Alto, CA, USA). A 5 μm, 200 A° polymeric C_{30} reverse-phase column (Pronto-SIL, MAC-MOD Analytical Inc., Chadds Ford, PA, USA) was used to separate the analytes. Initially, serum L and Z were quantified separately. Serum L levels (μmol/L) were added to serum Z levels (μmol/L) to create a combined serum L & Z value that was used in all analyses.

2.3.5. Neuroimaging Acquisition

MRI data were acquired using a General Electric Signa HDx 3T MRI scanner (GE; Waukesha, WI, USA). Images were acquired axially and covered from the top of the head to the brainstem. All slices were aligned to the anterior–posterior commissure line. Three-dimensional (3D) structural scans were collected using a high-resolution, T1-weighted fast spoiled gradient recall echo sequence (TR = 7.5 ms, TE = < 5 ms; FOV = 256 × 256 mm matrix; flip angle = 20°; slice thickness = 1.2 mm; 154 slices). The acquisition of the 3D structural scan lasted 6 min, 20 s. fMRI scans were collected using a T2-weighted single shot echo planar imaging (EPI) sequence (TR = 1500 ms, TE = 25 ms; 90° RF pulse; acquisition matrix = 64 × 64; FOV = 220 × 220 mm; slice thickness = 4 mm; 30 interleaved slices). Acquisition of the fMRI scans lasted 6 min, 33 s. Additionally, a pair of magnitude and phase images were acquired for use in fieldmap-based unwarping of the fMRI scans (TR = 700 ms, TE = 5.0/7.2 ms; FOV = 220 × 200 mm matrix; flip angle = 30°; slice thickness = 2 mm; 60 interleaved slices). The acquisition of the magnitude and phase images lasted 2 min, 20 s.

2.3.6. Data Analysis

fMRI scans were processed using Statistical Parametric Mapping (SPM12) [53]. Data were converted from GE DICOM format to NIFTI format using the dcm2nii conversion tool [54]. Pre-processing followed a standard procedure, including slice time correction to adjust for interleaved acquisition and realignment of the functional images to correct for motion. Fieldmaps were calculated from the acquired magnitude and phase images and applied to functional images to correct for distortion. Three-dimensional (3D) structural scans were co-registered to the functional scans and images were transformed into Montreal Neurological Institute (MNI) standard space. Deformation fields were created and applied to the functional images for spatial normalization to MNI standard space. Three-dimensional (3D) structural scans were segmented to separate brain tissue from cerebrospinal fluid, bone, non-brain soft tissue, and air. Images were smoothed using a 6.75 mm FWHM Gaussian filter.

Activation maps of JLO performance minus active baseline were created using the general linear model found in SPM12, with a statistical threshold of $p < 0.001$, family-wise error (FWE) corrected and a minimum of eight continuous voxels. These thresholds were chosen to balance between risk of Type

I and Type II error rates [55]. To assess the relationship between MPOD and neural activity within the hypothesized regions, a simple regression analysis was conducted, with the activation maps as the dependent variables and MPOD as the predictor variable. Analyses were repeated with serum L & Z as the predictor variable.

The relationship of L and Z concentrations with accuracy on the JLO task were evaluated in the Statistical Package for Social Sciences (IBM SPSS Version 21.0) using regression analyses, with measures of L or Z (MPOD or serum) as the independent variable and number of correct responses during the JLO condition as the dependent variable. Given that MPOD and serum L & Z were directionally hypothesized to positively relate to task accuracy, one-tailed statistical tests were conducted.

3. Results

3.1. JLO Behavioral Performance

Demographic and performance descriptive statistics can be found in Table 1. Due to a software error, performance data for the JLO task were lost for 11 participants. Of note, these participants did not significantly differ from the larger sample with regard to age, sex, education, mean MPOD, or mean serum L & Z concentration. MPOD ($n = 40$) did not significantly predict performance accuracy during the JLO condition, although results neared statistical significance ($R^2 = 0.07$, F = 2.841, $p = 0.05$). Similarly, serum L & Z ($n = 39$) also did not significantly predict accuracy during the JLO condition ($R^2 = 0.05$, F = 1.776, $p = 0.10$).

3.2. Whole-Brain Analysis

The JLO task minus active baseline contrast ($p < 0.001$, FWE corrected, minimal voxel cluster = 8) revealed widespread activation in regions commonly associated with vision, motor coordination, and visual–spatial decision-making, including the bilateral superior and inferior lateral occipital cortexes, right occipital pole, right occipital fusiform gyrus, right superior parietal lobule, bilateral paracingulate gyrus, left cingulate gyrus, bilateral middle frontal gyrus, bilateral frontal pole, bilateral precentral gyrus, bilateral insular cortex, and cerebellar vermis (see Table 2 and Figure 2).

Table 2. Whole-brain activation during the JLO task.

Region	x	y	z	Extent	T-Score
L superior lateral occipital cortex	−32	−88	12	35,624	23.75
L inferior lateral occipital cortex	−34	−88	2	*	21.38
	−38	−86	0	*	21.21
	−42	−64	12	*	20.35
R superior lateral occipital cortex	34	−80	22	*	21.63
	22	−64	52	*	21.58
	38	−78	12	*	20.03
	26	−72	36	*	18.76
	28	−74	30	*	18.40
R inferior lateral occipital cortex	34	−88	0	*	19.59
	38	−84	4	*	19.18
	40	−84	−4	*	18.52
R occipital pole	18	−96	6	*	18.81
R superior parietal lobule	32	−52	46	*	18.38
L cerebellum, vermis VI	−4	−72	−26	*	18.31
R occipital fusiform gyrus	38	−70	−10	*	18.06

Table 2. *Cont.*

Region	x	y	z	Extent	T-Score
R paracingulate gyrus	6	20	44	13,072	18.85
L paracingulate gyrus	−6	14	46	*	14.77
	−8	24	38	*	12.37
R middle frontal gyrus	28	0	52	*	17.54
	46	24	24	*	14.25
	50	30	28	*	13.01
L middle frontal gyrus	−26	−2	52	*	13.90
	−38	28	22	*	9.60
R insular cortex	32	20	−2	*	17.48
L insular cortex	−34	20	0	*	15.28
R precentral gyrus	42	6	28	*	17.15
L precentral gyrus	−32	−4	48	*	14.83
	−46	4	30	*	13.30
R frontal pole	44	44	−14	*	13.23
	38	58	0	*	11.16
	46	50	−8	*	10.16
L cingulate gyrus	−6	0	26	75	8.24
L frontal pole	−46	48	−4	30	8.05
	−48	44	−8	*	7.63
	−42	52	6	*	7.06

The table above reports whole-brain activation during the JLO task minus active baseline contrast ($p < 0.001$, family-wise error (few) corrected, minimal voxel cluster = 8). R = right hemisphere. L = left hemisphere. *x*, *y*, and *z* coordinates are in Montreal Neurological Institute (MNI) space (mm). * = cluster overlap with preceding row.

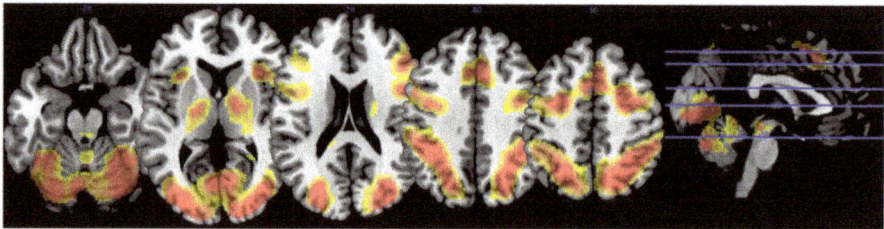

Figure 2. Whole brain activation during JLO task. The figure depicts brain activation during the JLO task minus active baseline contrast (independent of lutein and zeaxanthin levels). Activation superimposed on a single-subject anatomical template in MNI space provided by MRIcron [56]. To conserve space, only five slices were selected to showcase task-related BOLD response based on the largest extent activation.

3.3. Lutein and Zeaxanthin Analysis

3.3.1. MPOD

Following the JLO task, minus the active baseline contrast ($p < 0.001$, FWE corrected, minimal voxel cluster = 8), MPOD negatively predicted brain activity in regions associated with visual–spatial performance and decision-making, including the right superior and inferior lateral occipital cortexes, right angular gyrus, bilateral cingulate gyrus, right middle frontal gyrus, right frontal pole, right superior frontal gyrus, and right precentral gyrus ($p < 0.01$, see Table 3 and Figure 3). In other words, lower MPOD was associated with greater activation (i.e., "neural inefficiency") in these regions. As indicated in Table 3, the effect sizes for the relationship between MPOD and brain activation during the JLO task ranged from r = 0.343 to r = 0.403.

Table 3. Relationship between MPOD and brain activation.

Region	x	y	z	Extent	T-Score	Effect Size (r)
R superior lateral occipital cortex	54	−70	16	19	3.08	0.403
	56	−66	16	*	2.90	0.383
R inferior lateral occipital cortex	56	−68	12	*	2.94	0.387
R middle frontal gyrus	48	18	30	59	3.03	0.397
R frontal pole	0	60	16	31	2.93	0.386
L cingulate gyrus	−2	4	24	30	2.85	0.377
R cingulate gyrus	4	2	30	*	2.56	0.343
R angular gyrus	60	−50	38	15	2.84	0.376
	62	−50	34	*	2.81	0.373
R precentral gyrus	62	12	8	9	2.82	0.374
R superior frontal gyrus	6	56	25	10	2.62	0.351

The table above reports brain activation that was significantly and negatively associated with MPOD during the JLO task minus the active baseline contrast ($p < 0.01$). MPOD = macular pigment optical density. R = right hemisphere. L = left hemisphere. x, y, and z coordinates are in MNI space (mm). * = cluster overlap with preceding row.

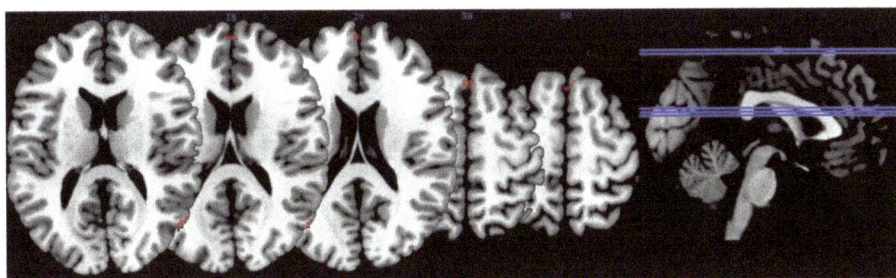

Figure 3. Relationship between lutein and zeaxanthin and brain activation. The figure depicts brain activation during the JLO task minus active baseline contrast that was significantly and negatively related to macular pigment optical density (MPOD) levels. In other words, individuals with lower levels of lutein and zeaxanthin showed an increased BOLD signal in these regions (i.e., "neural inefficiency). The activation is superimposed on a single-subject anatomical template in MNI space provided by MRIcron [56]. To conserve space, only five slices were selected to showcase task-related BOLD response based on the largest extent activation.

3.3.2. Serum L & Z

Serum L & Z also negatively predicted brain activity in regions associated with visual–spatial performance, motor coordination, and decision-making after subtraction of the active baseline ($p < 0.001$, FWE corrected, minimal voxel cluster = 8), including the bilateral superior lateral occipital cortex, left occipital pole, bilateral middle temporal gyrus, bilateral superior temporal gyrus, left superior parietal lobule, left planum temporale and planum polare, bilateral temporal fusiform cortex, left temporal pole, right posterior supramarginal gyrus, right lingual gyrus, left central opercular cortex, left parahippocampal gyrus, right thalamus, bilateral precentral gyrus, right postcentral gyrus, and left superior frontal gyrus ($p < 0.01$, see Table 4 and Figure 4). Thus, lower serum concentrations of L & Z were associated with greater activation and increased neural inefficiency in these regions. As indicated in Table 4, effect sizes for the relationship between serum L & Z and brain activation during the JLO task ranged from r = 0.360 to r = 0.492.

Table 4. Relationship between serum L & Z and brain activation.

Region	x	y	z	Extent	T-Score	Effect Size (r)
R precentral gyrus	16	−18	48	62	3.75	0.492
L middle temporal gyrus	−56	−8	−12	51	3.55	0.472
L superior parietal lobule	−36	−42	50	199	3.46	0.462
	−28	−56	58	*	3.29	0.444
L superior lateral occipital cortex	−20	−74	40	61	3.42	0.458
	−16	−88	36	12	2.73	0.381
R temporal fusiform cortex	36	−30	−16	33	3.36	0.452
L precentral gyrus	−20	−40	44	68	3.32	0.448
R superior lateral occipital cortex	26	−84	30	67	3.21	0.436
	24	−62	56	51	3.04	0.417
L superior frontal gyrus	−22	30	54	28	3.16	0.430
L posterior superior temporal gyrus	−60	−32	4	49	2.92	0.403
L planum temporale	−62	−22	6	*	2.70	0.377
L superior temporal gyrus	−52	−38	2	*	2.56	0.360
L occipital pole	−28	−96	6	9	2.99	0.411
L temporal fusiform cortex	44	−16	−16	9	2.95	0.406
R thalamus	24	−22	4	36	2.93	0.404
L planum polare	−36	−8	−10	19	2.87	0.397
R posterior supramarginal gyrus	46	−38	10	21	2.58	0.362
R posterior superior temporal gyrus	54	−36	8	*	2.87	0.397
L Heschl's gyrus	−46	−22	2	12	2.83	0.392
L parahippocampal gyrus	−32	−36	−18	22	2.83	0.392
R postcentral gyrus	6	−40	62	22	2.66	0.372
L central opercular cortex	−48	6	2	11	2.75	0.383
R anterior middle temporal gyrus	58	−2	−22	19	2.70	0.377
R anterior superior temporal gyrus	50	−2	−16	*	2.62	0.367
L temporal pole	−52	6	−18	10	2.67	0.373
R lingual gyrus	18	−60	−16	8	2.61	0.366

The table above reports brain activation that was significantly and negatively associated with serum L & Z during the JLO task minus active baseline contrast ($p < 0.01$). L = lutein. Z = zeaxanthin. *x*, *y*, and *z* coordinates are in MNI space (mm). * = cluster overlap with preceding row.

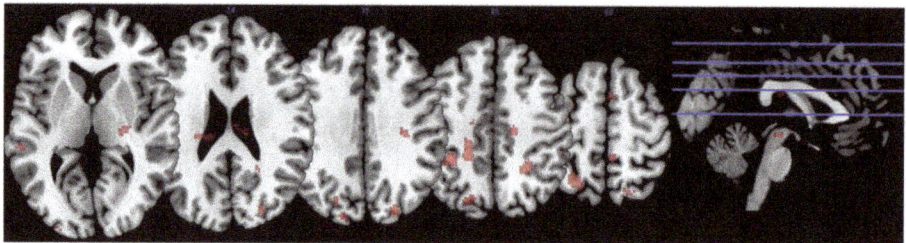

Figure 4. Relationship between lutein and zeaxanthin and brain activation. The figure depicts brain activation during the JLO task minus active baseline contrast that was significantly and negatively related to serum lutein and zeaxanthin levels. In other words, individuals with lower levels of lutein and zeaxanthin showed an increased BOLD signal in these regions (i.e., "neural inefficiency). The activation is superimposed on a single-subject anatomical template in MNI space provided by MRIcron [56]. To conserve space, only five slices were selected to showcase task-related BOLD response based on the largest extent activation.

4. Discussion

Although historically studied in relation to eye health [7], accumulating literature has demonstrated the potential for the xanthophyll, lutein (L), and its isomer, zeaxanthin (Z), to benefit a range of neurocognitive functions as well, particularly in older adults [2]. The present study is among the first attempts to investigate underlying neural mechanisms in vivo, using fMRI.

Initial whole brain analyses revealed a pattern of activation that is consistent with prior neuroimaging studies involving JLO and visual–perception more broadly, including occipito–temporal and parieto–frontal networks [40–42,57,58]. As hypothesized, both retinal (i.e., MPOD) and serum L and Z were negatively correlated with brain activity in several regions during JLO performance, though a somewhat different pattern of results was observed for the two measures. Although both MPOD and serum L and Z concentrations were associated with a BOLD signal in primary visual and spatial processing areas (e.g., lateral occipital cortex and occipital pole), a lower MPOD tended to more consistently relate to increased activation in frontal regions with demonstrated involvement in visual–perceptual performance, such as in the right superior frontal and right middle frontal gyri and the frontal pole [58,59]. Serum L and Z seemed to be more related to temporal–parietal regions associated with visual–spatial processing (e.g., the superior and middle temporal gyri, superior parietal lobule) in addition to primary visual areas. Thus, MPOD, which represents more stable L and Z concentrations acquired over time, may improve performance during visual–spatial tasks by increasing the efficiency of key frontal decision-making regions. In a complementary fashion, serum L and Z, which represent more acute dietary intake of nutrients, may improve performance by increasing the efficiency of visual–spatial processing.

It is not uncommon for the aging brain to show increased frontal involvement during cognitive performance, and consistent with the posterior–anterior shift in aging (PASA) model, this may reflect a form of compensation for age-related deterioration in other brain regions (e.g., occipitotemporal) [60]. Importantly, the compensatory PASA pattern has been specifically observed during visual–spatial perception and processing [61,62]. Individuals whose long-term dietary patterns include greater consumption of L and Z, as reflected by MPOD, may be especially buffered by general age-related neuropathological processes and thus require less frontal compensation. This interpretation is consistent with research demonstrating that older adults who can maintain healthy, "younger" brains (e.g., greater gray matter density) require less recruitment of additional neural circuitry (e.g., prefrontal areas) to carry out cognitive tasks relative to less successfully aging peers [63]. The ability to adequately complete a cognitive task with more focused cerebral involvement has previously been interpreted as "neural efficiency" [64] and seems consistent with the pattern observed here, likely due to the prophylactic effects of the L and Z carotenoids in neural tissue [65].

Although the precise role of frontal areas in the context of visuospatial performance remains to be fully elucidated, it has long been speculated to encompass a range of functions, such as decision-making, online maintenance of visual information necessary to make judgments, and more general cognitive control [58,66,67]. Observations in previous studies where "difficult" JLO items elicit prefrontal cortex activation, whereas "easy" items (e.g., those containing fewer line foils) do not have been interpreted as support for the possibility that complex visual–perceptual judgments require aspects of executive function [41,42]. Long-term dietary patterns involving L and Z intake, measured via MPOD, may improve the efficiency of neural processes underlying these higher order executive functions. Our findings are consistent with, and may help to explain, previous studies demonstrating a positive relationship between visual system ability and executive skills in older adults [68].

Contrary to expectations, L and Z levels were not significantly related to JLO accuracy in behavioral measures, although MPOD neared significance as a predictor. However, the findings were in the expected direction: individuals with higher MPOD and serum L & Z concentrations displayed relatively more accurate performances on the JLO task. Although there was a range in performance, accuracy on the JLO task (scores = 23–59), the overall mean accuracy was high (M = 52.53/60, SD = 4.49) with most participants scoring better than 87%. The high overall average could have a limited association with L and Z concentrations due to a "ceiling effect." Alternatively, or perhaps in combination, it is possible that an analysis with a larger sample and correspondingly greater statistical power would reveal a significant relationship.

Another explanation for the lack of significant correlation between L and Z concentrations and behavioral JLO performance lies in theories of compensatory aging, which suggest that there may be

Nutrients **2018**, *10*, 458

neural changes in the way older adults process information (e.g., recruitment of additional neural areas, increased neural activation) that allow them to maintain a high level of cognitive performance, and that nutritional factors contribute to these compensatory processes [69,70]. Our results showed that lower L and Z concentrations are associated with greater neural activation or neural "inefficiency" despite no statistically significant correlations with behavioral JLO performance. While older adults with lower L and Z concentrations appear to have maintained a high level of cognitive performance, they require greater compensatory neural activity than individuals with high L and Z concentrations. Thus, L and Z may contribute to "youthful" and efficient brain functioning regardless of cognitive outcomes.

A notable limitation of the present study is its cross-sectional nature, which prevents conclusions regarding the directionality of the observed association between L and Z and neurocognitive performance. Although findings from previous longitudinal studies have suggested that consuming carotenoids reduces the risk of age-related neurodegenerative diseases across time [71], only a few randomized controlled trials have evaluated the effects of L and/or Z supplementation in older adults [21,72]. As noted in recent reviews [73], additional randomized controlled trials are needed to determine whether low L and Z consumption contributes to declines in brain health and cognition or perhaps represents a consequence, such as poor nutritional choices resulting from cognitive impairments. In addition, the present study was restricted to a purely Caucasian sample that tended to be well educated and cognitively healthy. Replication in a more diverse sample is warranted to evaluate the generalizability of the observed findings.

Despite these limitations, the present study represents an important contribution to the literature and marks the first attempt to investigate neural mechanisms underlying the relationship between L and Z and visual–spatial functioning using fMRI. Findings suggest that L and Z may promote brain health and cognition in older adults by enhancing neurobiological efficiency in a variety of regions that support visual perception and decision-making. More broadly, the present study bridges the gap between the disciplines of nutrition and neuroscience to advance our understanding of the critical relationship between diet and brain function. Dietary features such as L and Z appear to hold considerable potential as modifiable and inexpensive lifestyle factors to promote neurocognitive health in the rapidly expanding older adult segment of the population.

Acknowledgments: The authors would like to acknowledge Joanne Curran-Celentano and Karen Semo for assistance with serum analysis. This work was supported by Abbott Nutrition, Columbus, OH, USA [research grant to LMRH, BRH, and LSM]; The University of Georgia's Bio-Imaging Research Center [administrative support to LSM]; and DSM Nutritional Products (Switzerland) who provided the supplements and placebos for the randomized-controlled trial from which the current data were derived.

Author Contributions: B.R.H., L.M.R.-H., and L.S.M. contributed to research study design; C.M.M., C.A.L., D.P.T., B.R.H., L.M.R.-H., and L.S.M. collected study data; C.M.M., C.A.L., D.P.T., and L.S.M. contributed to data analysis; C.M.M., C.A.L., T.L.R., and M.A.G. drafted the initial manuscript; C.M.M., C.A.L., K.R.J., B.H.R., L.M.R.-H., and L.S.M. primarily edited the manuscript; and C.M.M., C.A.L., T.L.R., M.A.G., D.P.T., K.R.J., B.R.H., L.M.R.-H., and L.S.M. assume responsibility for the final content of the manuscript.

Conflicts of Interest: The authors declare no conflict of interest. During a portion of data collection time, author L.M.R.-H. was employed by Abbott Nutrition while holding a joint appointment at the University of Georgia. BRH has consulted for Abbott Nutrition. No other conflicts of interest exist for the study authors, including C.M.M., C.A.L., T.L.R., M.A.G., D.P.T., K.R.J., and L.S.M. All statistical analyses were completed independent of the supporting agencies.

Registry Information: ClinicalTrials.gov number, NCT02023645.

References

1. Caracciolo, B.; Xu, W.; Collins, S.; Fratiglioni, L. Cognitive decline, dietary factors and gut–brain interactions. *Mech. Ageing Dev.* **2014**, *136*, 59–69. [CrossRef] [PubMed]
2. Johnson, E.J. Role of lutein and zeaxanthin in visual and cognitive function throughout the lifespan. *Nutr. Rev.* **2014**, *72*, 605–612. [CrossRef] [PubMed]
3. Craft, N.E.; Haitema, T.B.; Garnett, K.M.; Fitch, K.A.; Dorey, C.K. Carotenoid, tocopherol, and retinol concentrations in elderly human brain. *Exp. Anim.* **2004**, *21*, 22.

4. Johnson, E.J.; Vishwanathan, R.; Johnson, M.A.; Hausman, D.B.; Davey, A.; Scott, T.M.; Green, R.C.; Miller, L.S.; Gearing, M.; Woodard, J.; et al. Relationship between serum and brain carotenoids,-tocopherol, and retinol concentrations and cognitive performance in the oldest old from the Georgia Centenarian Study. *J. Aging Res.* **2013**, *2013*. [CrossRef] [PubMed]

5. Vishwanathan, R.; Neuringer, M.; Snodderly, D.M.; Schalch, W.; Johnson, E.J. Macular lutein and zeaxanthin are related to brain lutein and zeaxanthin in primates. *Nutr. Neurosci.* **2013**, *16*, 21–29. [CrossRef] [PubMed]

6. Ma, L.; Lin, X.-M. Effects of lutein and zeaxanthin on aspects of eye health. *J. Sci. Food Agric.* **2010**, *90*, 2–12. [CrossRef] [PubMed]

7. SanGiovanni, J.P.; Neuringer, M. The putative role of lutein and zeaxanthin as protective agents against age-related macular degeneration: Promise of molecular genetics for guiding mechanistic and translational research in the field. *Am. J. Clin. Nutr.* **2012**, *96*, 1223S–1233S. [CrossRef] [PubMed]

8. Feeney, J.; Finucane, C.; Savva, G.M.; Cronin, H.; Beatty, S.; Nolan, J.M.; Kenny, R.A. Low macular pigment optical density is associated with lower cognitive performance in a large, population-based sample of older adults. *Neurobiol. Aging* **2013**, *34*, 2449–2456. [CrossRef] [PubMed]

9. Renzi, L.M.; Dengler, M.J.; Puente, A.; Miller, L.S.; Hammond, B.R. Relationships between macular pigment optical density and cognitive function in unimpaired and mildly cognitively impaired older adults. *Neurobiol. Aging* **2014**, *35*, 1695–1699. [CrossRef] [PubMed]

10. Renzi, L.M.; Iannaccone, A.; Johnson, E.; Kritchevsky, S. The relation between serum xanthophylls, fatty acids, macular pigment and cognitive function in the Health ABC Study. *FASEB J.* **2008**, *22*. [CrossRef]

11. Vishwanathan, R.; Iannaccone, A.; Scott, T.M.; Kritchevsky, S.B.; Jennings, B.J.; Carboni, G.; Johnson, E.J. Macular pigment optical density is related to cognitive function in older people. *Age Ageing* **2014**, *43*, 271–275. [CrossRef] [PubMed]

12. Power, R.; Coen, R.F.; Beatty, S.; Mulcahy, R.; Moran, R.; Stack, J.; Howard, A.N.; Nolan, J.M. Supplemental Retinal Carotenoids Enhance Memory in Healthy Individuals with Low Levels of Macular Pigment in A Randomized, Double-Blind, Placebo-Controlled Clinical Trial. *J. Alzheimer's Dis.* **2018**, *61*, 947–961. [CrossRef] [PubMed]

13. Beatty, S.; Nolan, J.; Kavanagh, H.; O'Donovan, O. Macular pigment optical density and its relationship with serum and dietary levels of lutein and zeaxanthin. *Arch. Biochem. Biophys.* **2004**, *430*, 70–76. [CrossRef] [PubMed]

14. Hammond, B.R., Jr.; Wooten, B.R.; Smollon, B. Assessment of the validity of in vivo methods of measuring human macular pigment optical density. *Optom. Vis. Sci.* **2005**, *82*, 387–404. [CrossRef] [PubMed]

15. Burke, J.D.; Curran-Celentano, J.; Wenzel, A.J. Diet and serum carotenoid concentrations affect macular pigment optical density in adults 45 years and older. *J. Nutr.* **2005**, *135*, 1208–1214. [CrossRef] [PubMed]

16. Renzi, L.M.; Hammond, B.R.; Dengler, M.; Roberts, R. The relation between serum lipids and lutein and zeaxanthin in the serum and retina: Results from cross-sectional, case-control and case study designs. *Lipids Health Dis.* **2012**, *11*, 33. [CrossRef] [PubMed]

17. Nolan, J.M.; Stack, J.; Mellerio, J.; Godhinio, M.; O'Donovan, O.; Neelam, K.; Beatty, S. Monthly consistency of macular pigment optical density and serum concentrations of lutein and zeaxanthin. *Curr. Eye Res.* **2006**, *31*, 199–213. [CrossRef] [PubMed]

18. Akbaraly, N.T.; Faure, H.; Gourlet, V.; Favier, A.; Berr, C. Plasma carotenoid levels and cognitive performance in an elderly population: Results of the EVA Study. *J. Gerontol. Ser. A Biol. Sci. Med. Sci.* **2007**, *62*, 308–316. [CrossRef]

19. Lindbergh, C.A.; Mewborn, C.M.; Hammond, B.R.; Renzi-Hammond, L.M.; Curran-Celentano, J.M.; Miller, L.S. Relationship of lutein and zeaxanthin levels to neurocognitive functioning: An fMRI study of older adults. *J. Int. Neuropsychol. Soc.* **2017**, *23*, 11–22. [CrossRef] [PubMed]

20. Mewborn, C.M.; Terry, D.P.; Renzi-Hammond, L.M.; Hammond, B.R.; Miller, L.S. Relation of Retinal and Serum Lutein and Zeaxanthin to White Matter Integrity in Older Adults: A Diffusion Tensor Imaging Study. *Arch. Clin. Neuropsychol.* **2017**, 1–14. [CrossRef] [PubMed]

21. Lindbergh, C.A.; Renzi-Hammond, L.M.; Hammond, B.R.; Terry, D.P.; Mewborn, C.M.; Puente, A.N.; Miller, L.S. Lutein and Zeaxanthin Influence Brain Function in Older Adults: A Randomized Controlled Trial. *J. Int. Neuropsychol. Soc.* **2018**, *24*, 77–90. [CrossRef] [PubMed]

22. Zamroziewicz, M.K.; Paul, E.J.; Zwilling, C.E.; Johnson, E.J.; Kuchan, M.J.; Cohen, N.J.; Barbey, A.K. Parahippocampal Cortex Mediates the Relationship between Lutein and Crystallized Intelligence in Healthy, Older Adults. *Front. Aging Neurosci.* **2016**, *8*, 297. [CrossRef] [PubMed]

23. Walk, A.M.; Edwards, C.G.; Baumgartner, N.W.; Chojnacki, M.R.; Covello, A.R.; Reeser, G.E.; Hammond, B.R.; Renzi-Hammond, L.M.; Khan, N.A. The Role of Retinal Carotenoids and Age on Neuroelectric Indices of Attentional Control among Early to Middle-Aged Adults. *Front. Aging Neurosci.* **2017**, *9*, 183. [CrossRef] [PubMed]

24. Lezak, M.D. *Neuropsychological Assessment*, 3rd ed.; Oxford University Press: Oxford, UK, 1995; ISBN 978-0-19-509031-4.

25. North, A.J.; Ulatowska, H.K. Competence in independently living older adults: Assessment and correlates. *J. Gerontol.* **1981**, *36*, 576–582. [CrossRef] [PubMed]

26. Salthouse, T.A. Reasoning and spatial abilities. In *The Handbook of Aging and Cognition*; Craik, F.I.M., Salthouse, T.A., Eds.; Lawrence Erlbaum Associates: Hillsdale, NJ, USA, 1992; pp. 167–211.

27. Possin, K.L. Visual spatial cognition in neurodegenerative disease. *Neurocase* **2010**, *16*, 466–487. [CrossRef] [PubMed]

28. Hovestadt, A.; De Jong, G.J.; Meerwaldt, J.D. Spatial disorientation as an early symptom of Parkinson's disease. *Neurology* **1987**, *37*, 485–487. [CrossRef] [PubMed]

29. Raskin, S.A.; Borod, J.C.; Wasserstein, J.; Bodis-Wollner, I.; Coscia, L.; Yahr, M.D. Visuospatial Orientation in Parkinson's Disease. *Int. J. Neurosci.* **1990**, *51*, 9–18. [CrossRef] [PubMed]

30. Henderson, V.W.; Mack, W.; Williams, B.W. Spatial Disorientation in Alzheimer's Disease. *Arch. Neurol.* **1989**, *46*, 391–394. [CrossRef] [PubMed]

31. Ska, B.; Poissant, A.; Joanette, Y. Line orientation judgment in normal elderly and subjects with dementia of Alzheimer's type. *J. Clin. Exp. Neuropsychol.* **1990**, *12*, 695–702. [CrossRef] [PubMed]

32. Wahlin, T.-B.R.; Bäckman, L.; Wahlin, Å.; Winblad, B. Visuospatial functioning and spatial orientation in a community-based sample of healthy very old persons. *Arch. Gerontol. Geriatr.* **1993**, *17*, 165–177. [CrossRef]

33. Martin, A.D.; Stirling, W.J.; Thorne, R.S.; Watt, G. Parton distributions for the LHC. *Eur. Phys. J. C* **2009**, *63*, 189–285. [CrossRef]

34. Benton, A.L.; Varney, N.R.; Hamsher, K.D.S. Visuospatial judgment: A clinical test. *Arch. Neurol.* **1978**, *35*, 364–367. [CrossRef] [PubMed]

35. Benton, A.L. Constructional apraxia and the minor hemisphere. *Confin. Neurol.* **1967**, *29*, 1–16. [PubMed]

36. Benton, A.; Hannay, H.J.; Varney, N.R. Visual perception of line direction in patients with unilateral brain disease. *Neurology* **1975**, *25*, 907. [CrossRef] [PubMed]

37. Collins, D.W.; Kimura, D. A large sex difference on a two-dimensional mental rotation task. *Behav. Neurosci.* **1997**, *111*, 845. [CrossRef] [PubMed]

38. Paterson, A.; Zangwill, O.L. Disorders of visual space perception associated with lesions of the right cerebral hemisphere. *Brain* **1944**, *67*, 331–358. [CrossRef]

39. Gur, R.C.; Gur, R.E.; Obrist, W.D.; Skolnick, B.E.; Reivich, M. Age and regional cerebral blood flow at rest and during cognitive activity. *Arch. Gen. Psychiatr.* **1987**, *44*, 617–621. [CrossRef] [PubMed]

40. Fink, G.R.; Marshall, J.C.; Shah, N.J.; Weiss, P.H.; Halligan, P.W.; Grosse-Ruyken, M.; Ziemons, K.; Zilles, K.; Freund, H.-J. Line bisection judgments implicate right parietal cortex and cerebellum as assessed by fMRI. *Neurology* **2000**, *54*, 1324–1331. [CrossRef] [PubMed]

41. Kesler, S.R.; Haberecht, M.F.; Menon, V.; Warsofsky, I.S.; Dyer-Friedman, J.; Neely, E.K.; Reiss, A.L. Functional neuroanatomy of spatial orientation processing in Turner syndrome. *Cereb. Cortex* **2004**, *14*, 174–180. [CrossRef] [PubMed]

42. Tranel, D.; Vianna, E.; Manzel, K.; Damasio, H.; Grabowski, T. Neuroanatomical correlates of the Benton facial recognition test and judgment of line orientation test. *J. Clin. Exp. Neuropsychol.* **2009**, *31*, 219–233. [CrossRef] [PubMed]

43. Cabeza, R.; Grady, C.L.; Nyberg, L.; McIntosh, A.R.; Tulving, E.; Kapur, S.; Jennings, J.M.; Houle, S.; Craik, F.I. Age-related differences in neural activity during memory encoding and retrieval: A positron emission tomography study. *J. Neurosci.* **1997**, *17*, 391–400. [CrossRef] [PubMed]

44. Reuter-Lorenz, P.A.; Jonides, J.; Smith, E.E.; Hartley, A.; Miller, A.; Marshuetz, C.; Koeppe, R.A. Age differences in the frontal lateralization of verbal and spatial working memory revealed by PET. *J. Cogn. Neurosci.* **2000**, *12*, 174–187. [CrossRef] [PubMed]

45. Grady, C.L.; McIntosh, A.R.; Rajah, M.N.; Beig, S.; Craik, F.I. The effects of age on the neural correlates of episodic encoding. *Cereb. Cortex* **1999**, *9*, 805–814. [CrossRef] [PubMed]

46. Park, D.C.; Polk, T.A.; Park, R.; Minear, M.; Savage, A.; Smith, M.R. Aging reduces neural specialization in ventral visual cortex. *Proc. Natl. Acad. Sci. USA* **2004**, *101*, 13091–13095. [CrossRef] [PubMed]

47. Chee, M.W.; Goh, J.O.; Venkatraman, V.; Tan, J.C.; Gutchess, A.; Sutton, B.; Hebrank, A.; Leshikar, E.; Park, D. Age-related changes in object processing and contextual binding revealed using fMR adaptation. *J. Cogn. Neurosci.* **2006**, *18*, 495–507. [CrossRef] [PubMed]

48. Payer, D.; Marshuetz, C.; Sutton, B.; Hebrank, A.; Welsh, R.C.; Park, D.C. Decreased neural specialization in old adults on a working memory task. *Neuroreport* **2006**, *17*, 487–491. [CrossRef] [PubMed]

49. Morris, J.C. The Clinical Dementia Rating (CDR): Current version and scoring rules. *Neurology* **1993**. [CrossRef]

50. Levenson, J.H.; Kozarsky, A. Visual acuity change. In *Clinical Methods: The History, Physical, and Laboratory Examinations*, 3rd ed.; Walker, H.K., Hall, W.D., Hurst, J.W., Eds.; Butterworths: Boston, MA, USA, 1990.

51. Stringham, J.M.; Hammond, B.R.; Nolan, J.M.; Wooten, B.R.; Mammen, A.; Smollon, W.; Snodderly, D.M. The utility of using customized heterochromatic flicker photometry (cHFP) to measure macular pigment in patients with age-related macular degeneration. *Exp. Eye Res.* **2008**, *87*, 445–453. [CrossRef] [PubMed]

52. Wooten, B.R.; Hammond, B.R., Jr. Spectral absorbance and spatial distribution of macular pigment using heterochromatic flicker photometry. *Optom. Vis. Sci.* **2005**, *82*, 378–386. [CrossRef] [PubMed]

53. Ashburner, J.; Barnes, G.; Chen, C.; Daunizeau, J.; Flandin, G.; Friston, K.; Kiebel, S.; Kilner, J.; Litvak, V.; Moran, R.; et al. *SPM12 Manual*; Wellcome Trust: London, UK, 2014.

54. Rorden, C. DCM2NII (Version 7 October). 2007. Available online: http://www.cabiatl.com/mricro/mricron/dcm2nii.html (accessed on 14 October 2016).

55. Lazar, N. *The Statistical Analysis of Functional MRI Data*; Springer Science & Business Media: New York, NY, USA, 2008; ISBN 978-0-387-78190-7.

56. MRIcron Index Page. Available online: http://people.cas.sc.edu/rorden/mricron/index.html (accessed on 12 January 2016).

57. De Schotten, M.T.; Urbanski, M.; Duffau, H.; Volle, E.; Lévy, R.; Dubois, B.; Bartolomeo, P. Direct evidence for a parietal-frontal pathway subserving spatial awareness in humans. *Science* **2005**, *309*, 2226–2228. [CrossRef] [PubMed]

58. Ganis, G.; Thompson, W.L.; Kosslyn, S.M. Brain areas underlying visual mental imagery and visual perception: An fMRI study. *Cogn. Brain Res.* **2004**, *20*, 226–241. [CrossRef] [PubMed]

59. Biesbroek, J.M.; van Zandvoort, M.J.; Kuijf, H.J.; Weaver, N.A.; Kappelle, L.J.; Vos, P.C.; Velthuis, B.K.; Biessels, G.J.; Postma, A.; Utrecht VCI Study Group. The anatomy of visuospatial construction revealed by lesion-symptom mapping. *Neuropsychologia* **2014**, *62*, 68–76. [CrossRef] [PubMed]

60. Davis, S.W.; Dennis, N.A.; Daselaar, S.M.; Fleck, M.S.; Cabeza, R. Que PASA? The posterior–anterior shift in aging. *Cereb. Cortex* **2007**, *18*, 1201–1209. [CrossRef] [PubMed]

61. Grady, C.L.; Maisog, J.M.; Horwitz, B.; Ungerleider, L.G.; Mentis, M.J.; Salerno, J.A.; Pietrini, P.; Wagner, E.; Haxby, J.V. Age-related changes in cortical blood flow activation during visual processing of faces and location. *J. Neurosci.* **1994**, *14*, 1450–1462. [CrossRef] [PubMed]

62. Nyberg, L.; Sandblom, J.; Jones, S.; Neely, A.S.; Petersson, K.M.; Ingvar, M.; Bäckman, L. Neural correlates of training-related memory improvement in adulthood and aging. *Proc. Natl. Acad. Sci. USA* **2003**, *100*, 13728–13733. [CrossRef] [PubMed]

63. Düzel, E.; Schütze, H.; Yonelinas, A.P.; Heinze, H.-J. Functional phenotyping of successful aging in long-term memory: Preserved performance in the absence of neural compensation. *Hippocampus* **2011**, *21*, 803–814. [CrossRef] [PubMed]

64. Duverne, S.; Habibi, A.; Rugg, M.D. Regional specificity of age effects on the neural correlates of episodic retrieval. *Neurobiol. Aging* **2008**, *29*, 1902–1916. [CrossRef] [PubMed]

65. Sasaki, M.; Ozawa, Y.; Kurihara, T.; Noda, K.; Imamura, Y.; Kobayashi, S.; Ishida, S.; Tsubota, K. Neuroprotective effect of an antioxidant, lutein, during retinal inflammation. *Investig. Ophthalmol. Vis. Sci.* **2009**, *50*, 1433–1439. [CrossRef] [PubMed]

66. Kosslyn, S.M. *Image and Brain: The Resolution of the Imagery Debate*; MIT Press: Cambridge, MA, USA, 1996; ISBN 978-0-262-61124-4.

67. Miller, E.K.; Cohen, J.D. An integrative theory of prefrontal cortex function. *Annu. Rev. Neurosci.* **2001**, *24*, 167–202. [CrossRef] [PubMed]

68. Mewborn, C.; Renzi, L.M.; Hammond, B.R.; Miller, L.S. Critical flicker fusion predicts executive function in younger and older adults. *Arch. Clin. Neuropsychol.* **2015**, *30*, 605–610. [CrossRef] [PubMed]

69. Park, D.C.; Reuter-Lorenz, P. The adaptive brain: Aging and neurocognitive scaffolding. *Annu. Rev. Psychol.* **2009**, *60*, 173–196. [CrossRef] [PubMed]

70. Reuter-Lorenz, P.A.; Park, D.C. How does it STAC up? Revisiting the Scaffolding Theory of Aging and Cognition. *Neuropsychol. Rev.* **2014**, *24*, 355–370. [CrossRef] [PubMed]

71. Min, J.; Min, K. Serum lycopene, lutein and zeaxanthin, and the risk of Alzheimer's disease mortality in older adults. *Dement. Geriatr. Cogn. Disord.* **2014**, *37*, 246–256. [CrossRef] [PubMed]

72. Johnson, E.J.; McDonald, K.; Caldarella, S.M.; Chung, H.; Troen, A.M.; Snodderly, D.M. Cognitive findings of an exploratory trial of docosahexaenoic acid and lutein supplementation in older women. *Nutr. Neurosci.* **2008**, *11*, 75–83. [CrossRef] [PubMed]

73. Erdman, J.W.; Smith, J.W.; Kuchan, M.J.; Mohn, E.S.; Johnson, E.J.; Rubakhin, S.S.; Wang, L.; Sweedler, J.V.; Neuringer, M. Lutein and brain function. *Foods* **2015**, *4*, 547–564. [CrossRef] [PubMed]

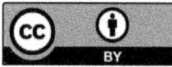

© 2018 by the authors. Licensee MDPI, Basel, Switzerland. This article is an open access article distributed under the terms and conditions of the Creative Commons Attribution (CC BY) license (http://creativecommons.org/licenses/by/4.0/).

MDPI

St. Alban-Anlage 66

4052 Basel

Switzerland

Tel. +41 61 683 77 34

Fax +41 61 302 89 18

www.mdpi.com

Nutrients Editorial Office

E-mail: nutrients@mdpi.com

www.mdpi.com/journal/nutrients

www.ingramcontent.com/pod-product-compliance
Lightning Source LLC
Chambersburg PA
CBHW051912210326
41597CB00033B/6123